Getting Golf Ready

An Introduction to Golf Fitness & Yoga for Golfers

by Kathy Ekdahl

Visit www.personalbestpersonaltraining.com for Kathy's Blog

Published by golfgurls.com
Design: Circle Graphics

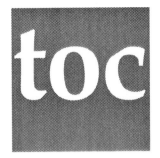

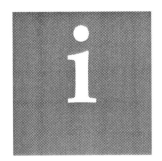

You are a dedicated golfer.

You buy the best equipment.

You take golf lessons every week.

You practice every aspect of your game religiously.

YET

You still have back and shoulder pain.

You still do not get the distance your clubs deserve.

You still get exhausted during your round.

Something is missing, isn't it?

What's missing is the physical conditioning
necessary to be the best golfer you can be!

Physical conditioning you ask? For golf? Why?

Proper physical conditioning is necessary because the golf swing is one of the most complex movements in all of sports, both explosive as well as a bit unnatural. The golf swing requires strong, flexible muscles to both produce and *withstand* the forces generated during the golf swing. Without this strength and flexibility, your swing will never reach its full potential, and your risk of injury is high. Unfortunately, most recreational golfers (perhaps you, or people you know?) take the physical aspects of golf for granted because of the slow pace of the game. The result: 1/4 to 1/3 of all golfers get injured while playing golf, with 40,000 trips to the emergency room each year (*Complete Conditioning for Golf.*) Women suffer more upper body injuries than men, but are less prone to back injuries than men. In general, the vast majority of injuries are from poor swing mechanics and a lack of physical preparation. And, of equal importance, most technical problems with the golf swing are closely related to a lack of proper strength, balance and flexibility. While your teaching pro will help you with swing mechanics, who guides you in understanding the physical changes you need to make to be a better golfer? Who advises you on how to remain injury free? Do you know what exercises are absolutely necessary for golf? Do you know which exercises will help, and which will hurt? Most likely not. But, you are not alone! The average recreational golfer does not have the expertise or knowledge to design golf specific exercise programs.

That's where we come in. As golfers, we understand your specific needs. We understand that you may not have a lot of experience with strength training, or understand what muscles are used during the swing and how to make them strong and flexible. Most golfers do not- no matter whether they are male or female.

But, rest easy. **Getting Golf Ready** will break down the components of a complete golf fitness program for you in easy- to-read sections so you can begin your journey to better golf and, better health.

So, let's get started!

Introduction to the Golf Swing

Golf fitness was a mere twinkle in the eyes of fitness trainers before Tiger Woods came along. Tiger Woods' exercise regimen transformed his body into the ultimate golf machine! Tiger matched perfect genetics with hard work—work that made him even more flexible and quick, and even stronger. Strong enough to withstand the pain of a torn ACL and *still* win a major championship. The exercise regimen he employed is not a secret—it is one that all of you can use to your advantage as well.

You can:

- Build core strength to translate power from the ground up to the club head

- Maximize flexibility for a complete swing

- Build strong muscles to enhance power and reduce injuries.

- Improve balance and coordination for uneven lies and proper weight transfer

Seems simple on the outside, but golf fitness necessitates a good understanding of the mechanics of the golf swing, and a better understanding of what aspects of fitness are necessary to enhance the golf swing. So let's start with an overview of the golf swing itself. Since I am not a golf pro, I'll speak in very general "layman's" terms. Let's all get on the same page....

The ADDRESS

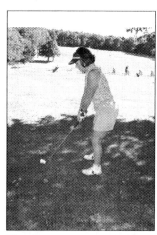

The golf swing begins at address. Knees are soft, with a slight forward bend from the hips, not the spine (spine needs to be in neutral alignment, ie straight), relaxed arms and head in neutral. This athletic position requires a strong core, so that the forward bend is from the hips, not the spine, and a strong upper back to prevent rounding of the shoulders and upper back. The hamstrings, located on the back of the thighs, must be flexible so that, again, the forward bend is from the hip space, not the low back. Bending forward from the hip, not the low back, is called "hip hinge" and is an essential aspect of the golf address. Tight hamstrings can hamper the ability to hip hinge and thus cause strain on the low back, a common problem with men.

The Address

Finally, good balance and body position awareness is key. Weight should be in the arches, not in the heels, with an even feel through the feet and ankles. Tight calves can hamper balance and body position, so this is another area to keep flexible.

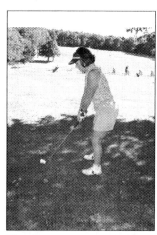

Correct

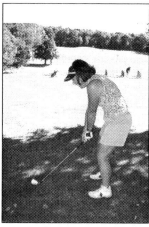

Incorrect

The BACKSWING

As you bring the club into your backswing, complicated changes occur throughout the body. Weight shifts to the back leg, but legs must remain relatively still, as the primary movement of the backswing is through a big torso turn. Torso rotation is the key to a good backswing, and if your flexibility is limited in the upper back and shoulders, a good turn is just not possible. Do you sit at a desk for work? Is your posture rounded forward? If so, then, chances are that your turn is inadequate. Tight chest muscles and anterior shoulders pull shoulders forward, rounding the upper back. This prevents optimal torso flexibility. This postural defect is called kyphosis, and is very common in women. I also often see it in people who lean over desks or computers for their jobs, who are not strong in the upper back, or who do not keep aware of posture.

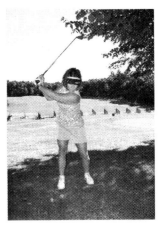

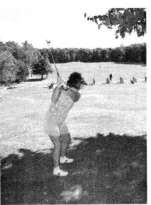

As the arms bring the club into the backswing, torso must turn, but legs must remain still. This causes power to be stored in the back hip (right leg if you are a righty) and core, power that will then be used on the downswing and ball strike. But, if your hips are tight or weak, the legs will move too much, causing power leaks (sways and slides).

Backswing

So, flexible, strong hips are a necessity for golf. Again, if you sit for your job, the likelihood is that your hips are weak and tight, not great for a good golf swing. As I mentioned previously, many people injure their upper bodies frequently in golf, and this is often a result of poor swing mechanics. You can't turn your shoulders because they are too tight, you can not store power in your hips because they are weak and tight, and thus you use your arms to try and power the club. See the connection?

The DOWNSWING and BALL STRIKE

At the top of your backswing, big things happen. Now, hips need to turn first, separating themselves from any movement of the upper body initially. This hip movement requires quick, strong hip rotation, something most women find very difficult. The ability to move hips separately from shoulders is called the X factor-

or coil- and this is what generates power. It is what makes pro golfers have lots of power in their swing and what allows them to whack the ball really far (a technical term!). Rest assured, it can be taught.

In addition, good shoulder flexibility and torso strength is key now to withstand the forces of the club as you come from the top of your backswing and strike the ball. At ball strike, great forces get translated into the wrists, elbows and shoulders.

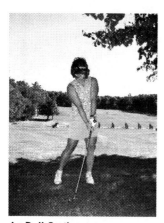
At Ball Strike

You need to be strong to withstand those forces. Good hand-eye coordination is essential at ball strike, but, more often than not, poor shoulder flexibility and torso rotation may already have the club on a poor swing path. Proper golf fitness techniques can address all of these issues.

At ball strike, weight is fully transferring from back leg to front leg and this is where all the power comes from. Your core and glutes (buttocks muscles) must fire with strength and speed. If glutes and core are not working optimally, you'll often feel pain in your low back because it is not well supported. Your glutes and abdominals hold the spine safely still at impact. Weak glutes and core will also prevent you from good weight transference and thus prevent you from striking the ball with the force you need to get good distance. That's not to say we need to crush the ball. Don't do it! As a former collegiate athlete, that was my big mistake- trying to crush the ball. Remember, the clubs are designed to do that for you. But, there is no club which can make a weak golfer a really strong one.

The FOLLOW THROUGH and FINISH

Once you have struck the ball, now your muscles need to slow down and eventually decelerate the high forces sent throughout your body. Your weight transfers to the front leg, moving through the ball strike. As muscles tolerate these forces, you still must keep a smooth swing to make sure you follow through. Strong upper back muscles, and in particular, strong shoulder and rotator cuff muscles, are necessary

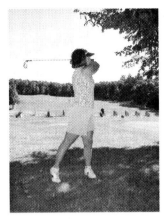

Follow Through

to prevent excessive strain on these areas during the follow through. A lack of proper follow through is once again related to torso flexibility, but also, balance. A lack of proper follow through will cause you to push or pull the ball. You must finish with weight on the outside of the front foot, "posting up," and this requires good ankle mobility, hip strength and balance.

So, now you can see how the physical body moves and changes through this complex movement that we call the golf swing. Swinging the club well, hitting the ball well, means being both flexible and strong. So, where do you start? What aspects of your physical fitness need help and what others are adequate? This is not an easy question to answer. I often have clients who come to me telling me they have poor flexibility because they are experiencing chronic pain in certain areas. But, things are not always as they seem! For example, someone may feel chronically tight hamstrings and assume this "feeling" means the hamstrings are too short- a flexibility limitation. However, in many circumstances, this actually means the hamstrings are weak or overworked. Hamstrings become overworked due to weak glutes, not because of shortened muscles. *Weakness* can cause muscle soreness, not just inflexibility. And, don't make the mistake the many of my clients initially made: assuming that your legs are strong because you walk or run. Walking, biking and running do not promote strength- only strength training does.

So, the question of where you start must begin with a physical assessment, usually performed by a TPI Golf Fitness Instructor or another educated strength and conditioning coach. But, secret revealed... *you* can perform a *self* assessment to give you the info you need to get started. Now, the fun begins.

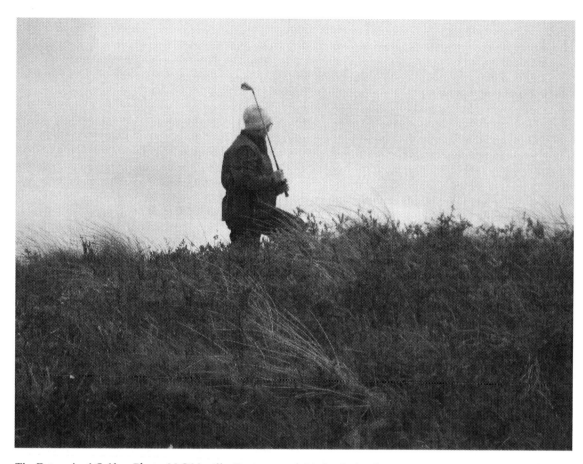

The Determined Golfer - Photo: N.C.Neville, Portmarnock Links, Ireland.

Chapter 2- Assess Your Own Golf Fitness

I'm sure that some of you may be thinking "Why do I need a fitness assessment, I am strong, look at my legs!" Or, "I have no injuries, no serious aches and pains, so things must be working fine, right?" I hear that all the time from my clients, the same clients who fail fitness assessments, who can't hit the ball more than 150 yards off the tee, or who hurt their backs lifting the laundry. How we look, or a lack of pain, are not ways to assess strength, flexibility and overall golf readiness. True strength, flexibility and balance have specific parameters- guidelines that tell us what is working well, what is not- and thus help steer us to the correct individualized fitness program. Further complicating things is the fact that we have become such a sedentary population. So much so, that many of the strong flexible muscles that we take for granted have become weak, tight or even shut off. Yes! Shut off! Glutes for example, are notorious for "shutting off" because we sit on them all day. Weak glutes, as mentioned previously, can cause back problems, hamstring injuries and a weak golf swing. Are your glutes strong? You'll never know until you test them objectively. (By the way, a big rear end does not always mean strong glutes, but a flat rear end often means weak glutes)

So, you... yes you... the one with the strong "looking" legs, the one who walks 4 miles a day... even you need a golf fitness assessment!

As we discussed in Chapter 1, the entire body contributes to a good golf swing. Everything from the calves, to the hips, to the shoulders, get involved. Thus, our self assessment needs to look at all of our joints, to assess their strength, their flexibility, their range of motion. The type of assessment you will be using is called a "Biomechanical Assessment", or a "Functional Assessment". You will perform an abridged version of the Titliest Performance Institute Golf Fitness Assessment, taught to TPI Certified Golf Fitness Instructors* around the world. In addition, I have added a few of my own assessments that I use with my personal clients. These are easy self assessments to help you identify your strengths or weaknesses in regards to flexibility, posture, balance and core and muscle strength.

(*The TPI Certified Golf Fitness Instructor Program is the most comprehensive golf fitness certification available, taught by the experts from Titliest's Performance

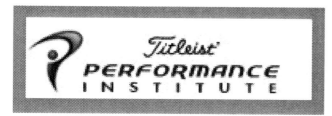

Institute, Dr. Greg Rose and Dave Phillips, pioneers in golf fitness. The TPI Certified Golf Fitness Instructor is educated in the latest research and development in the field of golf swing analysis, as well as techniques on how to assess, identify and overcome physical restrictions limiting a golfer's potential. The physical screening process and assessment is specific to golf, so that the TPI Certified GFI can then prescribe exercises, drills and golf fitness tips to overcome restrictions that affect the golf swing. Techniques used by TPI Certified GFI are applied to tour professionals and amateurs alike, and become the link between the golf pro and golf fitness.)

To prepare for the assessment, wear comfortable, loose clothes so that you can move freely. Not too loose- you need to be able to see your body. Take the test barefoot. You'll need to look at your feet for part of the assessment. As for equipment, you'll only need a golf club. No need to warm-up, you take the test in your "natural state"- whatever that may be. Have your assessment sheet and a pencil with you, so you can take notes on the test results. The results of the tests will determine what exercises are necessary to improve your golf fitness and overall health. You'll need to position yourself in front of a full length mirror for the test.

The Basic Rules:

- You should have no pain during any part of the assessment. Pain means stop the test immediately- and record a "fail" for that part of the test.
- The tests are graded as pass, fail or needs improvement. Be objective. Fail means fail, needs improvement means needs improvement. Don't confuse the two.
- The tests are performed without warm-up, without any preparation. They assess your body "as is".
- The assessment is not meant to diagnose or predict any injury, nor any medical condition ,so keep in mind this is a broad overview of your postural and biomechanical health.

This assessment is very general. User friendly. It's important you feel comfortable performing the tests, so don't worry, nothing is too complicated. I just want you to be aware of the important things you are going to learn about your body and how it moves. Understanding and awareness are the first steps to becoming a better golfer and a healthier you.

The Golf Fitness Assessments you will perform are:

- Postural Assessment
- Pelvic Tilt Test
- Overhead Squat Test
- Ankle Dorsiflexion Test
- Single Leg Balance Test
- Torso/Hip Rotation Tests
- Latissimus Dorsi Flexibility Test
- Shoulder Flexibility Test
- Gluteus Maximus (buttocks) Strength Test
- Hamstring Flexibility Test
- Quadriceps/Hip Flexor Flexibility Tests

Start with a Postural Assessment:

Your posture completely impacts your golf game from your set up to your ability to perform a complete golf swing. If you are hearing your mother's words, "Sit up straight!", you're getting the idea.

Look at yourself in the mirror.

Look at your posture from the side first. Is your posture straight, plumb line from crown of head down through hips, thighs and through feet? Or, are there unusual extra curves off set from this line? Normal spinal alignment does have some curves forward and backward (when observed from the side), but not excessive curves. In the normal spine, there is a slight forward curve of the neck, slight backward curve

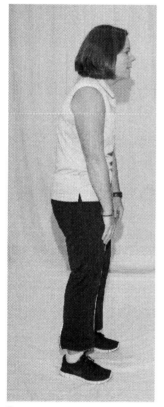

Poor posture

of the upper back, slight forward curve of the low spine. Notice how one curve direction alternates with the other? This is how your spine stays aligned.

So, let's look at your spine. For example, does your head jut forward? Are your shoulders back, chest up slightly- ideal posture- or are your shoulders rounded forward, chest caved in, so that your spine is shaped like the letter C? Does your lower back curve excessively forward or backward? Notice all these postures. If your upper back and spine curve backward like the letter C, you have a C shaped spine. C curves of the spine are problematic for golf, as they prevent adequate torso rotation during the back swing as well as prevent a full follow through and upright posture at finish. On the other hand, if your upper back curves normally, but your low back over arches forward, this is called lumbar lordosis, or S posture, and is a common cause of back pain during golf and during life. Tight hip flexors (located on the front of the hip and thigh) are one major cause of lumbar lordosis, as are weak abdominals. Luckily, we have exercises for those issues.

Next, look at your self from the front. Are your arms rotated inward, with the thumbs pointing at each other? This indicates tight shoulder internal rotators, and chest muscles, and weak external rotators. These are your rotator cuff muscles- the ones that you hear about that are so frequently injured during sports. But even abnormal daily posture of the shoulders and upper back can cause wear and tear to the rotator cuff, so this is an important observation. Shoulders should be back- thumbs pointing straight ahead. If your thumbs do point inward, you are in need of chest and front shoulder stretching, and rotator cuff and upper back strengthening to pull arms and shoulders into optimal alignment.

Lastly, observe if your shoulders are level, or does one shoulder drop lower than the other? Is one hip higher? Keep this in mind- it signals lateral imbalances that can eventually increase your risk for golf injuries. While front to back curves are normal in the spine, side to side deviations are not. If you notice excessive lateral deviations of the shoulders or hips, you may want to discuss this with your doctor.

Now look at your knees and feet. Do your knees turn in, or out, or do they face straight ahead? Knee caps should face forward, and, if they do not, it could be related to muscle imbalances that impact knee structure and mobility. It can also be congenital- but we can still do exercises to help prevent these abnormalities from getting worse from our own habitual posture and muscle imbalances.

Notice your feet. Is your weight primarily on the inside of the foot? This is called over pronation. Often, if the weight is chronically on the inside of the foot, the arch may fall. Do you have a good arch? Or, are you shifted to the outside of the feet? This is called over supination. Since all of your ground force must come through the feet during golf, having good ground contact and balance receptors is key. If your foot is not staying in neutral, this could impact your golf stance and thus, the swing as well.

Now that you have an idea whether you have any postural imbalances, you can choose exercises to improve posture. But, from now on, you need to consciously work to improve your posture on a day to day basis also. Pay attention when sitting or standing. When standing, chest up, shoulders relaxed, knees slightly bent, abs engaged, feet straight ahead with equal weight on both feet. Thumbs point straight ahead or even slightly outward, but not inward. When sitting, keep shoulders down and do not round forward from the upper back. Keep head and neck in alignment with the rest of the body, not jutting forward. If you work at a computer or desk for long hours, it is essential to get up and out of this unhealthy static posture at least once every hour. You should get up and do some of the stretches you will learn from this book.

Proper posture is the first key to a good golf game. If your posture is not optimal, your body can not move efficiently, and your golf swing will suffer. But poor posture impacts much more than sports. Habitual poor posture can become cemented. Muscles, tendons, ligaments and bones can become stuck in this abnormal posture and movement and overall function of the body is affected. Poor posture causes chronic pain, and can affect breathing and walking, much more important things than a good golf swing. So... as your Mom always said, "Sit up straight." She was right. Start now.

If you do nothing more than the above postural assessment, you have already learned so much about your body and your golf game. Later in this book, we will suggest stretches and strengthening exercises to help to correct the issues you discovered during your postural assessment. But, now, we will get more specific, as we assess your physical body joint by joint, looking for weakness, tightness, or poor movement skills.

This next part of the assessment is adapted from the TPI Golf Fitness Assessment, which is usually administered by a TPI Golf Certified Fitness Professional. Since you are self assessing, I've paired down the evaluation for you, the golfer, so that you can self test and discover how to create an individualized golf fitness program based on your own personal needs. Don't try and get too clinical or technical during the evaluation. Don't get caught up in passing or failing; don't let your ego drive the self assessment! More than anything, just observe how your body moves, where things feel tight, where things feel weak. And, lastly, note any feelings of discomfort or pain. If you have any pain during any part of the evaluation, stop immediately. Pain means you fail that part of the test. No worries- we are just information gathering.

Pelvic Tilt Test

You have already observed your natural standing posture, so you know what your inclination is as far as how you hold yourself erect. Let's look now at the low back specifically. The low back- also called the lumbar spine- should have movement that is normal and pain free. Often, from sitting or standing in poor posture, our normal neutral alignment can get lost. Our low back can then stop moving properly due to chronic weakness and tightness. Dysfunction, pain and injury can result.

Stand sideways to the mirror. Holding the golf club, get into your golf address. Then, drop the club, staying in golf posture, and cross your arms over your chest comfortably. Now, tilt- or should I say try and tilt your hips forward. In other words, tilt your hips so that the front of the hips tilt forward, back arches and buttocks lifts. Can you even do this? Do you have any movement at the low spine? Next, tuck your buttocks under, so that the front of the hips tilt back and low back rounds backward. (See photos below.) This is most likely easier, especially if you have a tendency towards C posture. Either way, your back should move in both directions, and the golf swing necessitates that you can tilt your hips forward- anteriorly, and backward- posteriorly. This test will follow your natural posture at

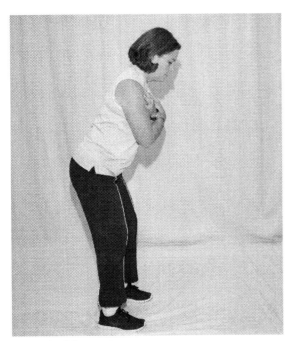

Hips tilted forward

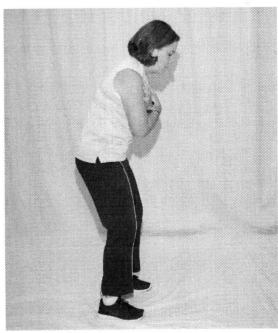

Hips tucked under

address. Those with a C posture won't be able to tilt the hips forward. On the other hand, if you have an excessive lumbar lordosis, as discussed previously, you won't be able to tilt the hips back.

The photos on this page show "Cat and Cow" yoga poses that demonstrate posterior pelvic tilt, hips tucked under (cat), and anterior tilt (cow), hips tilted forward. These are the same movements you performed standing, and may be easier for you to test if desired.

The experts at TPI have found that golfers with an excessive lordotic posture are more likely to injure their backs during golf. Remember - the best lumbar posture for golf address is a neutral one - buttocks neither tucked under, nor sticking out.

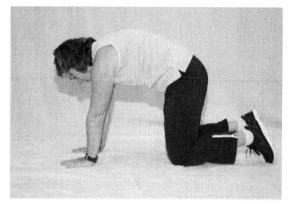

Cat Spine

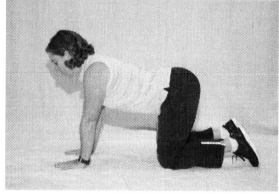

Cow Spine

Overhead Squat Test

This is the most challenging test, as you will be asked to perform a squat. The human body is designed to squat. A good squat tells us everything is working perfectly. However, if you have physical limitations to performing a squat such as current knee, hip or back injuries- skip this test. And, remember, as with all tests, any unusual pain, and the test should stop. It's a fail.

Stand with your feel hip width apart, feet pointed straight ahead or slightly out-*slightly*. Holding a golf club in your hands, with hands wider than shoulders, raise your arms over your head, elbows straight. This is the first part of the test. If you can not raise your arms directly over your head easily, with elbows straight, then your shoulders and upper back are too tight. If the arms are forward of your head, or elbows are significantly bent, or if you are leaning back, this doesn't count. It's just your body trying to compensate for the tightness. Note now if this is happening.

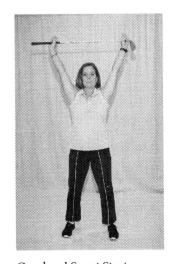

Overhead Squat Start

Next, keeping arms over head, sit BACK into heels (still keeping toes on ground) and squat down, lowering buttocks as far down as you can. Optimally, this would be below your knees. Keep spine upright, arms overhead, heels down completely. If you cannot come close to performing the squat shown in this photo, record a "fail." If you can not squat and maintain this erect posture, it means torso and back muscles are too tight, core is weak. Often you will also feel tightness and discomfort in the shoulders and mid and lower back. This should tell you something. Now, if you can not squat without heels lifting, this could indicate overly tight calf muscles. Or, if you can squat down, but can not get buttocks low enough, this often means weak abdominal and buttocks muscles. Keep notes on your findings. If your squat is not quite low enough, or you fold forward during the squat, record "needs improvement."

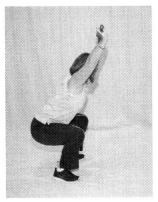

Overhead Squat

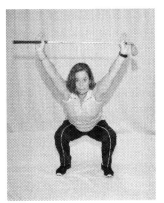

Overhead Squat Front

Ankle Dorsiflexion Test

It may seem strange that we are evaluating the ankles. But, the feet give us great feedback about balance and weight shift during the golf swing. Ankles which do not flex properly, whether due to a previous injury, or just chronic tightness, will impact your golf swing as well the overall health of your knees, hips and back. Everything is attached. This is called Kinetic Chain. Abnormalities at any point in the kinetic chain, from the head to the feet, can alter posture and function along other parts of the chain as well.

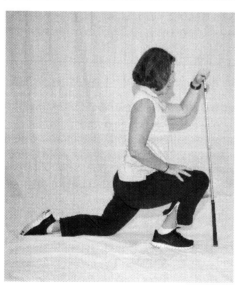

Ankle Dorsiflexion Test Start

Kneel on one knee, forward foot flat on the ground, knee directly over foot with the shin perpendicular to the floor. Keeping the heel *completely on the ground,* push the knee of the forward leg as far over your toes as possible. The knee should be able to jut 4 inches in front of the toes. (To measure 4 inches, you can position yourself with your foot 4 inches from the wall or another vertical measure like a yard stick or golf club)

This means optimal ankle dorsiflexion, a key to good lower body function. Perform the test on both ankles. If you can not press the knee 4 inches forward of the toes *while keeping the heel down,* then you have poor flexibility of the calf muscles. We can stretch these muscles! Also note — If you were unable to squat, and you fail this test as well, this could be a major contributor to your failed squat.

Ankle Dorsiflexion Test

Single Leg Balance Test

Professional golfers can stand on one foot for over 20 seconds **with their eyes closed.** Balance is a very important part of golf. As you move the club from backswing to follow through, the club, and your body's momentum, changes your balance.

You need to be able to "feel" when your weight is forward, or back, where the weight is on your feet, and you must be able to keep balance as you swing through the ball. At finish, your weight is on the front foot, knee locked and posted up. This takes good single leg balance! Balance is not just about your feet however. Good balance is also a function of a good core. So, this test is not just about your feet or ankles, but about your hip and core stability we well.

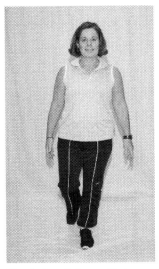
Single Leg Balance Test

Stand on one foot. Lift the other leg up, without it touching the standing leg. Hold still and tall for as long as possible, keeping track of how many seconds you can balance (use a clock with a second hand). If you wobble terribly- test is over. Don't try and regain balance and keep time if you almost fall over. Perform the test on both legs. Is there a discrepancy? Note this. It has a big impact on your golf swing, and thus your entire game. If you can not hold single leg balance for more than 10 seconds or so, you really need work on your core and hip stability. *And we did not even perfrom the test with the eyes closed!* If you can stand on one leg for 20 seconds, try the test with eyes closed as well. Very enlightening. Again, note which leg is more stable, imagine how that would impact your golf swing, and your overall potential for slips and falls.

Your foot placement during this test, (as noted in the postural assessment) also plays a role here. Does your foot generally roll in? This is pronation, and, sometimes, it can be improved with hip strengthening and some stretching. Or, does your foot generally roll out? This is supination. A challenging problem for some, myself included. Not so easy to fix. Walking or standing on the outside of the feet, or the inside of the foot for that matter, can cause ankle, knee and hip problems up the Kinetic Chain, so keep this in mind.

Torso/Hip Rotation test

This is where you'll get a real understanding of how well your body moves during the golf swing. As discussed previously, the torso needs to be able to move independently of the hips, and vice versa. Poor flexibility, or poor core stability, can prevent the two parts from separating, and this will greatly impact your golf swing, and the power you can generate during your golf swing.

Stand at address, as you did during the pelvic tilt test. Cross your arms over your chest. First, try and rotate your shoulders without moving your hips whatsoever.

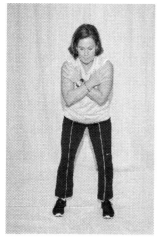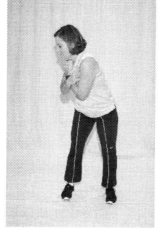

Shoulder Rotation Test

Can you do it? If your hips move, it may mean your chest and upper back muscles are tight. It could also mean your core is not strong enough to stabilize the hips. We'll explain this further in a moment.

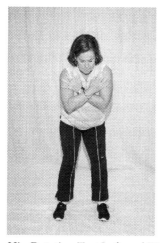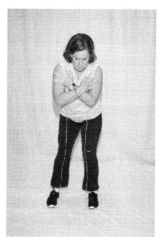

Hip Rotation Test Left and Right

Next, try keeping the arms and torso perfectly still and rotate only the hips. Think Elvis Presley, or the twist, but not slide and sway, which we often see in the golf swing when hips are tight. This part of the test is difficult for most people. If this is true for you, it could mean the hips are too tight, your core is weak, or that this movement pattern- hip internal and external rotation- is unfamiliar to your body. Let's investigate this further-as it is the hallmark of a strong powerful golf swing.

Try this: grab your club and place it in front of you upside down, holding on to the club head. Push down slightly so you stabilize your upper body. Now, try and rotate the hips. If you can do this, then you have the movement pattern, you have the flexibility, but it is your *core* stability that is lacking. If you still can not rotate the hips- then it may be a flexibility or neuromuscular patterning issue, and we can work on this! Later, we'll discuss in more specifics how to assess and correct hip rotation, but for now, just get a sense of how well your hips move.

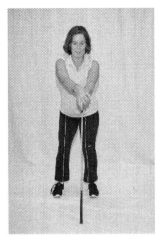

Club Assisted Hip Rotation

Let's investigate your shoulder turn- ie torso rotation – a bit further. A good golfer has at least 45 degrees of rotation of the torso. 60 degrees or more is even better. While this is often measured using a device called a goniometer, you can get a ballpark idea of your torso flexibility with a self test. Sit in a chair with your knees together. Put a pillow between the knees to insure that you do not rotate the low back during this test. Place the golf club behind your back, holding it across your shoulders. Stop…. Is this painful or difficult? It should not be. If so, you know that your chest and anterior shoulders (part of the rotator cuff) are too tight. If this is uncomfortable for you, place the club in the front of your body with arms crossed over it. The test can also be done as in the photo, with

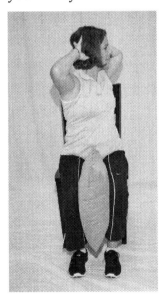

Seated Shoulder Rotation

hands behind the head, but make sure torso rotates and not just elbows and head. But, take note of this. Stretching the chest and shoulders is essential for you to prevent injury and improve your golf swing.

Now, sit up tall, and rotate your shoulders to one direction. This should feel good-it is a good stretch! But, that aside, for the test, notice how far you can turn. Then, rotate to the other side and compare the two. It is not uncommon for the golfer to be assymetric. Which direction can you turn farther? If you can turn right (and you are a righty) this corresponds to your back swing. Pretty important to have full range of motion here- 45 degrees or more-or you'll try and get range of motion with your low back, or a change in golf posture- and this can put you at risk for back injury, or poor swing mechanics. Important note: The low back should not be the primary source of rotation during the golf swing. Rotation comes from the upper spine and then the hips. This is why proper torso rotation and hip rotation are necessary to prevent back injury during golf.

Note whether you can twist farther to one direction than the other.

Latissimus Dorsi Flexibility Test

This assesses one of the large muscles that attaches at the upper back, lower back

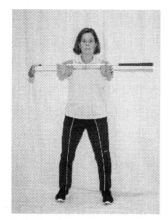

Lat Test Start

and back of the shoulders also called the "lats." The lats, when too tight, can create rounded posture and result in an incomplete golf swing. The good news- the lats are easy to stretch! To perform the test, go to a wall, and stand with your back against it. Bend your knees and drop down until you are in a half squat. Press low back against wall, shoulders and head against the wall as well..... if possible? If you have significant postural issues, you may find your back is too arched, or your head and shoulders do not touch the wall.

If you note any of these issues, the test can not be performed properly due to the postural abnormalities, so skip this and record a "fail." If you are close, keep going. Now, raise arms in front of you with straight elbows and thumbs pointed up. You

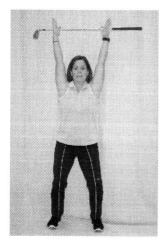

Lat Test Top

can place a golf club between the thumb and pointer finger so it is parallel to the floor if you wish, or you can do this without the club. Raise arms up over head, elbows straight, and try and touch wall with thumbs. You should be able to do this easily. If not- if your shoulders lift up, or elbows bend, or your low back arches off the wall- note this. It means your lats are too tight and need work. The "lats" are a prime mover during the golf swing. These muscles take a lot of stress during a round of golf. If they are tight or weak, injury is possible.

Shoulder Flexibility Tests

Good range of motion at the shoulder joint is essential for a good golf swing. The shoulders should be a highly mobile area, and if movement is hindered by tight muscles, injury can and will result. While we assessed the tightness of the major muscles of the torso with some of our previous tests, we also need a specific test for the shoulders. Shoulder rotation is performed by a group of muscles called the Rotator Cuff muscles. Generally, these muscles hold the arm bone in the shallow socket of the shoulder girdle. Every time we swing a

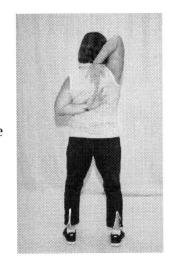

Rotator Cuff Flexibility Test

golf club, or throw a ball, the momentum of the swing/throw is putting stress on these muscles. They need to be strong, and we have exercises to strengthen the 4 rotator cuff muscles, but they also need to be flexible. This is because, as mentioned above, another of their roles is to rotate the arm bone outward, like at the top of the backswing and at finish. Tight rotator cuff muscles mean greater stress on these comparatively small muscles during golf. Not a good thing. To check the rotation of your shoulders, bring one hand over head, and bend the elbow, dropping your hand down to your upper back, palm down. Bring the other hand behind your back at waist height, palm up, and try and reach up your back to touch the fingers of the over head hand. Optimal shoulder rotation would be demonstrated by the fact be that you can touch the finger tips of both hands together. Are you laughing right now? I know. Most of my clients have at least a 6 inch space between finger tips when they first come to see me. (This is often due to poor posture, slouching, extended desk work, rounded shoulders.) Perform the test on both arms. Note which shoulder has better flexibility. If you experience any pain, stop the test and note this. An inability to reach up with the lower hand means that most likely, the rotator cuff muscles at the back of your shoulder are not 100%. During the next portion of the shouder flexibility test we will look further at the external rotation of the shoulder (performed by the rotator cuff muscles) with a very simple visual test.

Stand tall and bring one arm out to the side, elbow and shoulder in alignment, parallel to the floor. Bend elbow to 90 degrees. Now, keeping your elbow from dropping, rotate arm up as far as you can so palm faces forward. The hand should

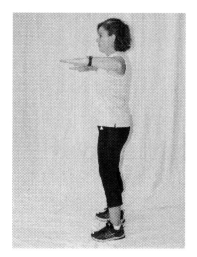 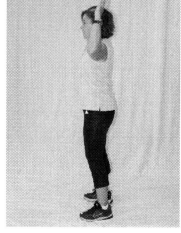 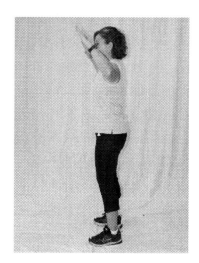

Rotator Cuff Test Start   Rotator Cuff Test Normal   Rotator Cuff Poor Rotation

easily rotate behind the elbow. Do not lean back as you rotate. Do both arms and note any assymetry. A right shoulder deficiency affects your backswing (if you are right-handed), a left shoulder deficiency affects your follow through. Either way, these deficiencies put you at risk for a shoulder injury from golf.

Gluteus Maximus (buttocks) Strength Test

The buttocks muscles are one of the most important muscle groups to keep strong for a powerful golf swing. The gluteus maximus, also called the glutes, is a core muscle that provides stability for the back and provides power and speed in all sports. Yet, many people have very weak glutes from sitting on them all day, or from not properly training them. When the glutes are weak, typical injuries occur to nearby muscles like the low back muscles or the hamstrings, as these muscles overwork to compensate for the weak glutes.

To test the strength of the glutes, lie on your back with both knees bent and feet flat on the floor, hip width apart. Keep toes pointed straight ahead, not outward. Bring your arms up straight over your chest and put palms together (note that in the photos below I have my arms at my side. It is better to have the arms up over your chest). Now, hike your hips up into the air. This is called a bridge. Next, straighten one leg out so that the leg is parallel to the floor, not up in the air. Hold this position for 10 seconds. The glute of the leg that is on the floor has to contract to hold you in the bridge. If it is not strong, a cramp will result in your hamstring, or your hips will drop lower and lower over the course of the 10 seconds. A hamstring cramp is a fail immediately, as is any back pain. Shaking or lowering of the hips and leg means the glute is weak, but still working. Do both legs. Note any asymmetry, as it is not uncommon for one side to be stronger than the other.

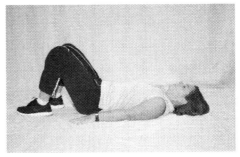

Buttocks Strength Test

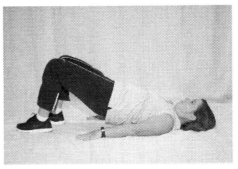

Buttocks Test Mid - (Supine Bridge)

Hamstring Flexibility Test

The hamstrings are located on the back of the thigh, attaching the leg to the pelvis at the top of the thigh, and inserting below the knee at the top of the calf. Tight hamstrings are very common, especially in men, or anyone who sits a lot during the day. Tight hamstrings can also cause postural abnormalities like rounding of the lower back, a no-no for your golf address, and tight hamstrings can lead to back pain. To assess the flexibility of your hamstrings, lie on your back, legs straight out in front of you on the floor. Lift one leg up, keeping the knee perfectly straight. Make sure the non tested leg stays flat on the floor, as does your low back. You should be able to bring the leg to a 90

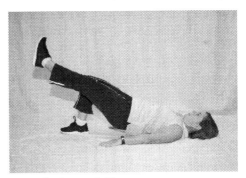

Buttocks Strength Test

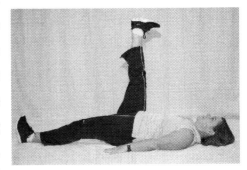

Hamstring Flexibility Test

degree angle at your hips. In other words, your leg should be able to be straight over your hips without strain. If the hamstring is very tight, it may only get to 45 degrees, which is indicative of significant tightness that needs to be addressed!

Hip Flexor/Quadriceps Flexibility Test

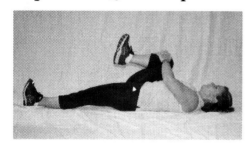

HF Test Normal

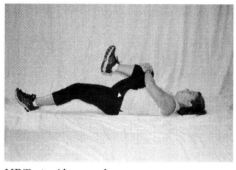

HF Test - Abnormal

As I have mentioned countless times, sitting is truly the nemesis of the human body. Hip muscles get very tight and shortened, due to sitting for extended periods of time. The front of the hips get especially tight, and this tightness can cause knee and hip pain and dysfunction eventually. Two muscle groups we need to assess are the hip flexors, which attach the thigh to the hip itself, and the quadriceps, which is located along the front of the thigh.

There are several ways to check the flexibility of your hip flexors, but one of the easiest is called The Modified Thomas Test. Lie on your back with both legs straight on the floor. Pull one knee into your chest, holding it just below the knee. Normal hip flexor flexibility means the leg on the floor remains completely flat while the other leg is bent into the hip. If the straight leg raises off the floor, that hip flexor is tight. Repeat the test on the other side as well.

Another simple test I use is just a kneeling hip flexor stretch. Kneel on one knee, as in the ankle dorsi flexion test, front foot flat on the floor with a vertical shin, with the thigh of the kneeling back leg perpendicular to the floor, toes curled under. Squeeze the glute of the kneeling leg, pressing the thigh forward, while keeping the lowback straight, not arched at all. If you have a hard time pushing that hip/thigh forward and feel significant stretch in the front of the hip, then you are tight. Tight hip flexors mean stress on the back and are a sign of weak abdominals as well, thus

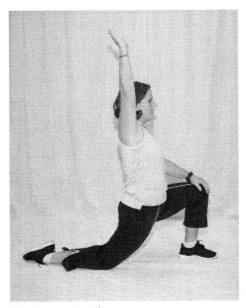

Hip Flexor Stretch

increasing back injury risk. You'll notice in the photo to the left that my arm is up in the air. This is not necessary for the test, but is a wonderful part of the stretch to correct poor flexibility in the hip flexors.

To test the flexibility of the quadriceps muscle, lie on your side with knees bent slightly. Grab the foot of the leg that is on top, gently pulling heel in towards buttocks. The thigh should stay aligned or slightly behnd the hip bone. The heel should come all the way into the buttocks. Keep back still. You should have no back pain with this test, and if you do, stop immediately.

If you can not pull the heel into the buttocks, then your quadriceps muscle group (which is also part of your hip flexor muscle group) is tight. The remedy for this tightness is easy- just do this test as a stretch.

You've finished the assessment. You made it! While there are other tests that are available to us to gain more information about our physical golf

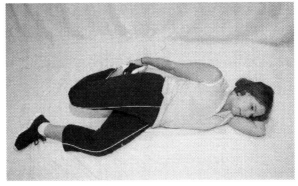

Quadriceps Flexibility Test

readiness, these are the basics. We've looked at the flexibility, mobility and strength of almost all of your major muscle groups. Now, we can take this information , whether it be pass, fail or needs improvement, and design a golf fitness regimen that is individualized for your body. The following chapters will outline the exercises you need to perform to correct any weaknesses or imbalances you found during the assessment.

Chapter 3 - Creating Your Customized Golf Fitness Program

Now that you have completed your golf fitness assessment, it is time to compile this information and create a customized golf fitness program. As you have learned in the previous chapters, there are many aspects of fitness that impact your golf game. From flexibility, to strength, to balance, to core strength and stability, we need to address all of these fitness components in order to create a balanced fitness program and consequently, a balanced body.

Before we begin however, one aspect of fitness "programming" that you need to first consider is your personal schedule. As a fitness trainer with over 23 years in the industry, I have seen many fitness enthusiasts who create a wonderfully complete exercise program only to discover that it takes them 2 hours a day to do it! You can have the most impressive exercise program in the world, but if your schedule does not allow time to execute it, frustration and feelings of failure can over ride all your great intentions. So, it is important to consider how much time you want to spend on fitness. For overall good health, most people need an hour a day to undo their sedentary life styles. If this is not possible, start smaller. Shoot for 1/2 hour- 45 minutes a day, 3 days week. For golf fitness (and general fitness) this is a great place to start. We know through years of scientific research, that to improve any aspect of fitness, it must be worked on 2-3x/week. Any less, and you won't see improvement. Keep in mind, golf fitness and general fitness cross over quite a bit, so your fitness program can address both types of fitness at once.

The next few chapters will address different components of golf fitness. I highly recommend that you address all aspects of golf fitness: flexibility, core strength (also referred to as core stability) whole body strength and balance. But, as we discussed above, I realize that not everyone may have the unlimited time to do so. This is why the self assessment is so important. Rather than wasting time on exercises that may not be a top priority, we now have the ability to prioritize your fitness needs based on the results of your assessment. The assessment actually is designed to highlight the areas of fitness you most need help with. For example, you may have noticed that you passed all the flexibility tests, but failed the strength tests. This would mean you need to emphasize strength versus flexibility. Or, you may be fine with the lower body tests, but failed the upper body tests. Whatever the findings, at least we now have direction!

Before we move on to the chapters on each individual aspect of fitness, I think it is a good idea to quickly review the definitions of golf fitness we are using in this book. They may be a bit different than traditional fitness components, and your complete understanding is most important.

The components of golf fitness we are addressing are:

Flexibility- the ability of your joints and their attachments to move smoothly and freely through their normal range of motion. Various joints have greater ranges of motion and more complex movement capabilities than others, but there are norms we should try to achieve in order to move well and prevent injury and chronic pain. Not only does each individual joint have "norms", it is also important to realize that tightness in one area can cause injury in another. For example, the hips and ankles have the ability to move in multiple directions. The knee does not. Poor flexibility in the hips or ankles could thus cause knee pain and injuries. Shoulders are also highly mobile and need to retain good flexibility, but because the bony structure of the shoulders is very delicate compared to the hips, shoulders also need a lot of support from the bigger muscles of the torso. Shoulders that lose flexibility due to bad posture or desk work and do not have good muscular support from the strength of the torso muscles, are prone to injury during golf. And, poor flexibility in the shoulders (and upper back) could result in elbow pain, low back pain and neck pain. Everything is attached, and everything impacts the rest of entire body.

Core Strength (also referred to as Core Stability)- the strength of all of the muscles that attach to the spine in order to support and stabilize the spine during movement and during static postures such as sitting at a desk or addressing a golf ball. For our purposes, I am separating out core strength/stability from whole body strength, although there is a huge crossover. I am doing this so you can understand what I believe are the most important muscles to get stronger for golf and for life. For example, I'd much rather see you work on the strength of your upper back or abdominals, than waste time on working on your biceps and triceps. It is just a matter of priorities. While arm strength is important for golf, arm strength can not undo the damage a weak core does on you golf game.

Whole Body Strength- the ability of the muscles of the body to do work and to support the bones during sports activities or daily activities that require movement of the body itself or heavy external loads. For golf, strength has everything to do with power and ball flight distance, but of equal importance, good strength is a key to injury prevention. You could be the most flexible "Gumby" in the world, but if you are weak, you still can get injured due to the repetitive stress of the golf swing. For women, this is frequently a major cause of injury. While women generally are more flexible than men, they need to balance flexibility with good strength. And yet, time and again, I hear from women (and men) that they do not want to do too much strength training because it can make them "muscle bound". This is one of the biggest myths not only in golf fitness, but in general fitness as well. Strength training rarely, if ever, makes a woman muscle bound. Genetically, we just do not have the testosterone to make that kind of muscle bulk. Even in men, strength training should not hamper the golf swing UNLESS the man is not addressing flexibility. Unfortunately, this is all too common in men. And, as we discussed earlier, since men generally need more flexibility work than women anyway, this is a recipe for disaster when it comes to golf. There also is a big difference between doing work to get stronger, and doing work to get "bigger." It is possible to get stronger without building huge muscles. Personally, I added 20 yards of distance by improving my strength without any detriment to my flexibility because I actually stretch after my workouts. Imagine that!

Balance- a very important aspect of golf fitness that is actually a compilation of core strength/stability and good flexibility. Good balance is a key to preventing falls and injuries, and moving well in active recreational sports such as soccer or running. For golf, good balance is necessary for a proper golf swing, especially on uneven lies. Even on the tee box, poor balance manifests itself as poor weight transference and a poor finish. Many people assume that balance is only related to the muscles of the calves and ankles. But balance really starts with our center of gravity- known to you as *the core*. So, while proper ankle and foot alignment is a part of balance, it is just one component that contributes to good balance. (Note- balance is also a factor of your eyesight and your vestibular system- the "balance wheel" located in your inner ear. Also, balance can be affected by neurological conditions and aging itself, which unfortunately we can not control. However, we can and should still try and improve balance even under these conditions)

Now, there are other areas of fitness that are also essential to good health that we did not address in your golf fitness assessment. They are: cardiovascular endurance and nutrition (this includes hydration). We will briefly discuss them later, but let's just suffice it to say that good nutrition and hydration is essential for our fueling during golf, a game that traditionally lasts quite awhile compared to most sporting events and games. And, obviously, good cardiovascular (and muscular) endurance goes a long way to helping us golf as well on the 17th hole as we did on the 3rd.

Now that we are all on the same page, let's start by looking at your flexibility first.

Chapter 4 - Flexibility

It's common knowledge that optimal flexibility is important for golf. Yet, even with our sedentary lifestyles and lots of sitting for work or relaxation, most people do not make adequate time to stretch. And, when we do, we often stretch the wrong muscles. Luckily, flexibility is not hard to improve. It can take as little as 5-10 minutes a day to improve the flexibility of the tight areas we discovered during your assessment. There are many different types of exercises which can improve flexibility. Even strength training has been shown to improve flexibility. Primarily, we will perform two types of flexibility exercises:

Static Stretches- held for a long duration of time designed to relax tight, short muscles. These are the stretches that most of us are familiar with.

Dynamic Flexibility- flexibility gained through repeated controlled movements that mimic the movements used during the sport or exercise. For example, a kicker in football will kick repetitively before a field goal to lengthen the hamstring muscle before the kick. Or, a golfer will swing a club prior to the round to promote good upper body shoulder flexibility.

Both types of stretches have their pluses and minuses.....

Static stretches tend to be safer, but may not be appropriate before golf. Research has shown that static stretching before a round of golf decreases power output, distance and accuracy during the round.[1] Static stretches are best done after golf, or on a daily basis as a regimen to improve flexibility over time.

Dynamic stretching (or dynamic flexibility) is the best method for improving flexibility before a sporting event (Golf) or workout. Dynamic flexibility lengthens muscles without shutting them down, like static stretching does. It makes sense that dynamic stretching would be important before a sporting event as we want our muscles to be activated, not calmed down or shut down. However, dynamic stretches may not be the best way to improve flexibility over time, and caution needs to be taken when performing these exercises as not to overdo a movement and strain a muscle.

Thus, you may find that your golf fitness regimen has both dynamic and static stretches depending on the goal or timing of stretching. Later in this book, we will outline golf warm-ups and cool-downs, and you will see that most pre- golf stretches should be dynamic and most post golf stretches, or day-to -day stretches, will be static.

So, get out your golf fitness assessment sheet. Depending on the results of the assessment, we will recommend stretches to address your areas which need better flexibility. The tests that addressed flexibility during the assessment are:

Pelvic Tilt Test
Ankle Dorsiflexion Test
Torso/Hip Rotation Tests
Latissimus Dorsi Test
Shoulder Flexibility tests
Hamstring Flexibility Test
Quadriceps and Hip Flexor Flexibility Tests

[1] Journal of Strength and Conditioning Research, Gergley JC, "Latent Effect of Passive Static Stretching on Driver Clubhead Speed, Distance, Accuracy and Consistent Ball Contact in Young Male Competitive Golfers", December 2010-Volume 24-Issue 12 pp3326-3333

Some general notes about stretching......

I've given you a variety of stretches to choose from for each tight area. No matter what type of stretch you choose, you must use perfect form. If possible, perform the stretches initially in front of a mirror so you can assess your posture and form. Except where noted, your back needs to stay straight during the stretches. Often, when stretching, you will inadvertently contort your posture to make the stretch easier. Try to avoid this- it makes the stretch less effective and can cause pain or injury to other areas of your body.

It is best to have the muscles slightly warmed up before you begin stretching. Warm muscles respond best to stretching. Cold muscles will not respond well, and you could injure yourself if not careful. A warm up could be a brief walk, a few dynamic stretches, or, my favorite, foam rolling. Foam rolling is also called "self myofascial release" (also called SMR for short). SMR involves using various tools like rollers, balls or sticks to self massage muscles and fascia. Fascia is the thin tissue that covers muscles and is thought to play a great role in chronic pain. Fascia can become tight and compress muscles and nerves and cause pain. Both stretching and a proper warm-up will help to release tightness of the fascia as well as tightness of the muscles and their attachments. If you are not familiar with self myofascial release tools, you can use your hands to massage tight tissue, but I highly recommend you investigate these techniques. For me, it has been a Godsend to relieve the occasional pain I get from exercise, sitting, and, life in general. As much as I'd love a daily massage, it's not feasible, and self massage is a great way to get my tissue healthy at no cost.

When performing daily static stretches, I recommend you hold the stretches 30 seconds, and repeat the stretch 2-3 times per body part. Take the stretch to mild discomfort and breath. Steady, slow breathing signals the muscles to release and relax. Holding your breath causes muscle tension, so pay attention to your breathing. (This is very important to do on the golf course as well. Holding your breath on the tee box, or during a challenging shot, can cause muscle tension in areas that you need to relax, like shoulders, arms and hands.)

If your assessment suggests dynamic stretches, these stretches are held only briefly, if at all, but repeated 5-8x per area. Again, perfect form is necessary, and, since the stretch is achieved through movement, pay attention to keeping movements in control. Do not bounce or throw the body part with momentum. As with any stretch, you should not have pain. If you feel anything other than normal stretch pain, stop immediately.

Pelvic Tilt Test- This first test is an important one to evaluate the motion of the lumbar spine, the low back. During the golf swing, your back needs to be able both flex and extend to create a safe and powerful swing. You also need to have good awareness of "neutral" spine- the ideal position for the low back during your golf set up. However, with excessive sitting, lack of exercise, or habitual poor posture, we often lose sight of what "neutral spine" is, and our low backs may assume a posture that is either overly flexed, known as "C" spine, or overly extended, known as lumbar lordosis.

Your spine should be able to curve as the hips tuck under (flexion), and extend as the buttocks is lifted back and the hips tilt forward (extension). During the test, if these motions were not easy or natural, then your back does not have normal motion. To address this deficit, I recommend "Cat and Cow", a yoga movement performed on all 4's. If your spine naturally assumes a "C" spine, you need to work on Cow- extension of the spine. If your spine is naturally over-extended with a large curve at your low back, emphasize Cat- flexion of the spine.

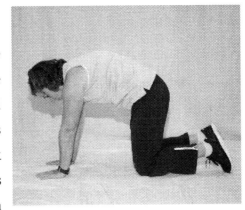

Cat

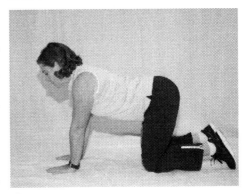

Cat and Cow- Dynamic. Repeat 8-10x until spine feels fluid and relaxed. Great for pre golf. Cow

Ankle Dorsiflexion Test- This test looks at the motion of the ankle joint as related to the flexibility of one of the calf muscles, the Soleus muscle. The Soleus muscle attaches to the foot via the Achilles Tendon, and a tight Achilles Tendon and Soleus muscle can cause ankle and foot pain and dysfunction. Injuries such as ankle sprains, Achilles Tendonitis and Plantar Fasciitis are often caused by a tight, inflexible calf and Achilles. Tight calf muscles prevent good movement at the ankle joint and will affect your golf game in many ways – from "feel" when addressing the ball, to walking the course, to balance and even power output. An inflexible ankle joint can prevent a good squat motion, so this can be one cause of a poor Overhead Squat Test as well.

If you could not reach your knee 4 inches over the toes when performing the test, the stretches you should perform are:

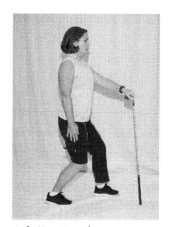 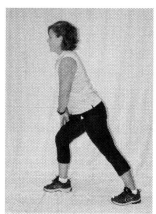

Achilles Stretch   Standing Calf

Static Calf Stretches against the wall- both straight knee and bent knee. (Straight knee will stretch the upper calf muscle called the gastrocnemius)

Torso/Hip Rotation Test This test had two parts. Just like your golf swing, the test separated rotation of the torso from rotation of the hips. In previous chapters, I detailed how important it is for us to be able to separate rotation of the shoulders and upper body from rotation of the hips in order to store power in our hips, and to avoid rotation of the low back, which can cause injury and pain. It is very important to realize that the low back should NOT be the source of rotation during our golf swing. But, an inflexible upper spine or tight hips can force our bodies to try to get rotation from the lumbar spine. Our upper spine/ torso is designed to have 60 degrees or more of rotation. Our lumbar spine is only designed to have 12-14 degrees of rotation, and it will be very unhappy if asked to do more!

If you could not rotate your shoulders without moving your hips, this is an indication of EITHER tight upper back muscles OR, a weak core which fails to hold the rest of the body still during upper body rotation. For now, let's just address poor upper body rotation. Exercises to address this deficit are:

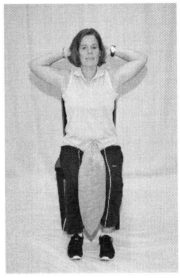

Seated Twist Start

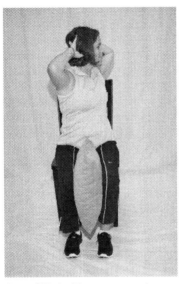

Seated Twist Turn

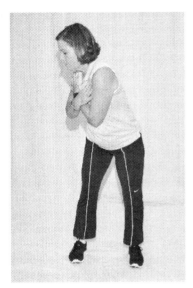

Standing Torso Twist

Seated Twist- Dynamic and Static

Standing Torso Rotations-Dynamic.

Lying Side Twist- Static (a yoga pose) best done static

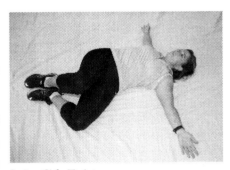

Lying Side Twist

If you could not rotate your hips separate from your torso during the second portion of the test, again, this could indicated EITHER poor hip internal and external rotation OR a weak core. To differentiate this, I demonstrated the same test while holding on to the top of the golf club while trying to rotate hips. Did you try this? If you CAN rotate the hips while pressing down on the golf club, then a weak core may be somewhat at fault. But, even if you can improve hip rotation while doing this, my experience with almost all my golfers is that most of them have poor hip rotation as well. So, we still need to address this.

Next are dynamic and static stretches to improve internal and external rotation of the hips. For golf, internal rotation is absolutely crucial to a proper golf swing, yet most people are unaware of this essential aspect of hip motion.

Dynamic

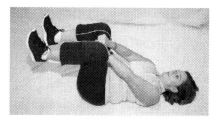

Windshield Wipers - Start

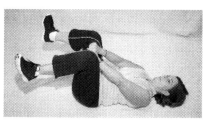

Windshield Wipers - Finish

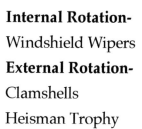

Internal Rotation-
Windshield Wipers
External Rotation-
Clamshells
Heisman Trophy

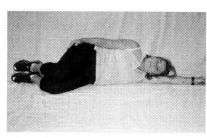

Clam Shell -Start

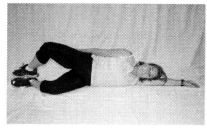

Clam Shell -Mid

Static
Seated Cross
Legged Hip
(also called
90/90 stretch)-
This stretch can
also be done

standing on the golf course, or lying on the floor in "Cradle" yoga pose.

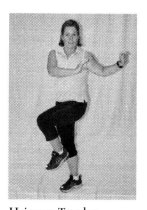

Heisman Trophy

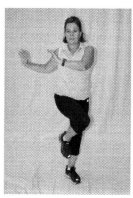

Heisman Trophy

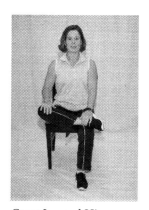

Cross Legged Hip

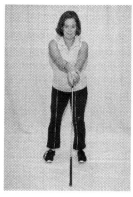

Standing Hip Rotation

To keep things simple, you can also just practice the movements as in the test. Standing hip rotations (the test- with or without club assist)

Latissimus Dorsi Flexibility test

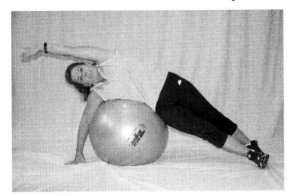

Physio Ball Lat Stretch

The Latissimus Dorsi muscles (the "lats") are large muscles that attach the arms to the torso, run along the sides of the back and attach at the low back. They do take up quite a bit of room on the back itself. The lats pull the arms down into the sides, an integral part of the golf swing. The lats also need to be very strong to help the body create and then withstand the forces of the golf swing, which can reach speeds of up to 100mph. Tight lats pull shoulders forward and create bad posture- a real no-no for golf. Normal length lats allow the arms to reach overhead easily, which is what we evaluated during the test. If you could not reach the arms easily over head, if the thumbs could not touch the wall easily, then you need to stretch your lats with the following stretches:

Club Assisted Lat Stretch
Physio Ball Lat Stretch
Side Stretch

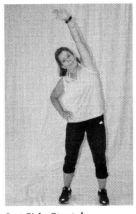

Lat Side Stretch

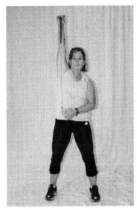

Lat Stretch With Club

Shoulder Flexibility Test

As I've mentioned before, the shoulders are a highly mobile joint. Good flexibility is part and parcel of how the shoulders are designed to be used. (Note I said "good" flexibility. We don't want over flexible shoulders either. This can cause joint instability and serious injury.) Shoulders- and I am using this term broadly right now- can get very tight from sitting, work, poor posture and injuries. Shoulders, in fact, are very prone to injury; they are most common body part injured during weight training. When I say shoulders, I am primarily referring again to the rotator

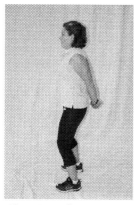

Chest Stretch

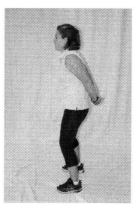

Chest Stretch - Incorrect

cuff muscles at the back of the shoulder. But I also want to highlight the front of the shoulders- where the chest muscles attach at the arms and up towards the neck. Tight chest muscles contribute to rounded shoulders and a "C" spine, and combined with a weak or tight rotator cuff, are a recipe for disaster. Tight chest muscles prevent good torso rotation. If you cannot easily place your hands behind your head as if to twist, this is one indication that your chest is too tight. (This is one reason why you cannot hold a club behind your back to warm-up. That, and tight rotator cuff muscles) So, I am going to include some chest stretching here as well.

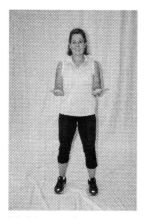

No Money - Start

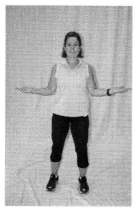

No Money - Finish

During the test, if you could not clasp your hands behind your back, or you could not rotate your arms up towards 90 degrees, you need to do the stretches pictured on this page, the chest stretch, no money, and the rotator cuff stretch.

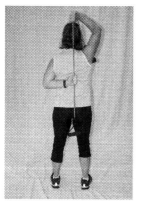

Rotator Cuff Stretch

To perform the rotator cuff stretch using a rope or tie, put your hands into the test position, using the tie to bridge the gap. Never force this stretch. Gently pull both up, to stretch the front of the lower arm, and down to stretch the lats and triceps of the upper arm. Reverse arms and repeat.

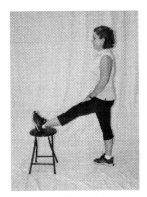

Hamstring Flexibility Test

Hamstring Flexibility Test

Of all the tests, most women pass this one easily, while men are often very tight in this area. Overall, I see more chronic tightness as most people are sitting for extended periods of the day for work. If you passed the test, or came close, this does not mean you never need to stretch them, it's just that this area will not be your top priority. If you have chronic pain in your hamstrings, yet your flexibility is normal, this commonly can indicate a weak buttocks muscle. The hamstring has to over work make up for the buttocks not doing its job well enough. The pain from an overworked hamstring can mimic the pain from hamstring tightness. This is why this test is so helpful, whether you pass or not.

If you could not lift your leg to 90 degrees, perpendicular to the ground, your hamstrings need stretching. You can perform:

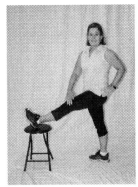

Standing Hamstring
With Rotation - Start

Standing Hamstring
With Rotation

Standing Hamstring
    with Rotation- static
Lying Hamstring- static
Down Facing Dog- static
Leg Swings- dynamic

One last note- I have not given you either a standing toe touch or a seated toe touch. I am not a fan of these stretches because they involve rounding of the

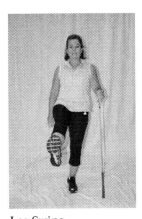

Leg Swing

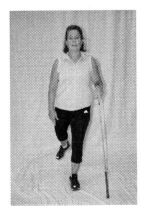

Leg Swing

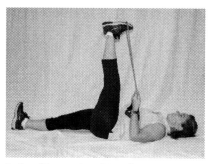

Lying Hamstring Stretch

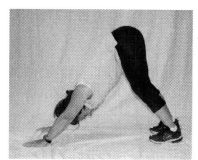

Down Facing Dog

low back to achieve the stretch. Standing toe touch is especially problematic if you do not or can not "hip hinge" (we discussed this earlier in chapter 1 in regards to your golf set up). I'd rather see you do a single leg stretch with a neutral spine.

Quadriceps and Hip Flexibility Tests-

The hip flexor muscle group is located on the front of the hip and thigh and is responsible for pulling the knee up towards the chest. Excessive sitting causes the HF to become short, and this can cause problems with back pain, hip and thigh pain as well as knee issues. Tight hip flexors will also shut off the core from working properly. This can be a big problem when it comes to golf, as your core is the center of your power (and back health). One of the hip flexors runs downs the front of the thigh to the knee and is considered one of the quadriceps muscles, also on the front of the thigh. Stretches for the quad and hip flexor are similar and there is some cross over.

Regarding the quadriceps test, if you could not easily pull your heel back into your buttocks, you need to do the following stretches shown on the next page:

Side Lying Quadriceps Stretch
Standing Quadriceps Stretch

These stretches will also lengthen the hip flexor muscle group to some extent, but more work is necessary usually.

In the second part of the test, you laid on the floor with one knee into your chest. If the other thigh is not pressed flat to the floor, the hip flexor of that leg is too

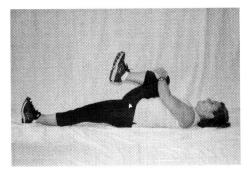

Hip Flexor Stretch - Normal

tight and needs additional work. Also, if you could not kneel on one knee with the thigh of that leg at a 45 degree angle and the low back straight, then again, your HF needs work.

To stretch the hip flexors- merely do these tests- Hold the stretch statically.

There are dynamic stretches for both the hip flexor and quadriceps, but we will save these for our golf warm-ups which we will cover in chapter 8.

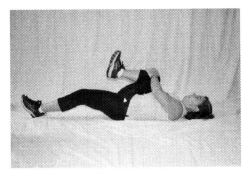

Hip Flexor Stretch - Abormal

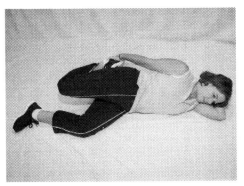

Side Lying Quadriceps

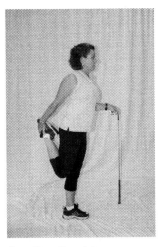

Standing Quadriceps

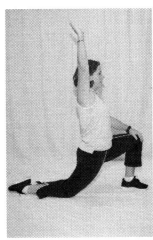

Hip Flexor Stretch

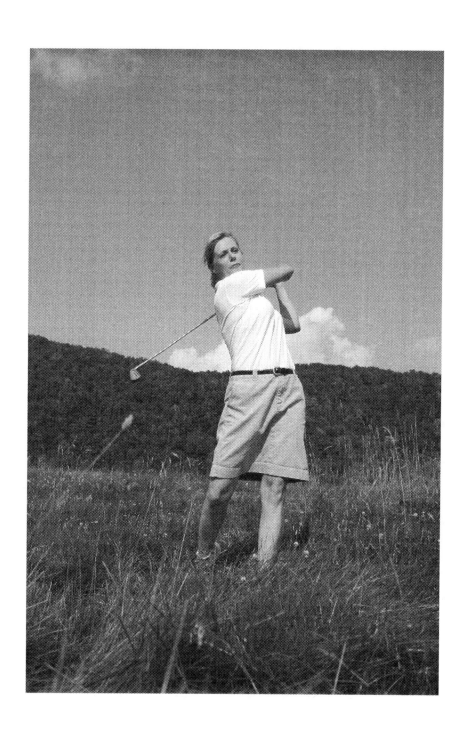

Chapter 5- Core Strength and Stability

As few as 15 years ago, a millisecond in "scientific research time", very few people, other than exercise science researchers, understood the important role that "The Core" plays in how we carry ourselves, how we move, how we do work, or stay safe during sports and play. Strength training programs, up until the early 1990's, emphasized form over function. Big, bulky muscles, the goal of most strength training programs in the old days, were created through a series of exercises that isolated each muscle to enhance its form. There was no greater emphasis on strengthening the glutes or abdominals(major muscles of the core), than on each individual head of the triceps. In fact, extraordinary amounts of time were deliberately spent on getting the biceps or triceps or shoulders to "look a certain way". Strength training thus meant "bodybuilding." By the late 1990's, both the scientific community, as well as fitness professionals, were beginning to realize that bodybuilding did not produce the best athletes, nor the fittest neuromuscular system. Bodybuilding did not teach our bodies the movement skills they needed; the ability to move well, to move freely, without injury or pain. In the 1990's, back and shoulder injuries from strength training were at an all time high. We were really missing something!

That something turned out to be "The Core". ..A buzz word that permeates every exercise regimen, every infomercial, every fitness magazine. And, even since that first "aha" moment- the realization that training the core properly reduces injuries and produces better athletes- we have continued to evolve our definition of core strength and stability. When I say we, I mean the medical community, the fitness community, the sports performance training community. Unfortunately, most average exercisers and recreational athletes have not evolved with us. They still think that a crunch is the best way to work the abs, or that abdominal and low back nautilus machines are fine for core strength. In fact, these methods are as outdated as bodybuilding, and, often, just as risky.

So- what exactly should we do to improve the strength and stability of the core? Well, it depends on an individuals' daily activities and stressors such as sports, work, and even sitting. Golf, for example, puts very specific stress on the spine. Analysis of the golf swing shows that with club head speeds reaching up to 100mph, the stress on the body in some areas is equivalent to the stress put on a football player's body during body contact in a football game! Good core strength is the only way we can produce and withstand the forces generated during golf.

(Complicating things is the fact that many recreational golfers spend a good amount of their day sitting for work. As we discussed previously, sitting for extended periods of time shuts off important core and postural muscles. Thus, we arrive on the first tee with shut down muscles and poor postural awareness. This is why a proper golf warm-up is as essential as all other aspect of golf fitness. See Chapter 8 for great golf warm-ups.)

Specifically, during various parts of the golf swing, our core needs to:

-Hold the spine still at address

- Hold the hips still on the takeaway

- Create power in our hips and glutes on the downswing

- Translate power at impact and protect the spine at impact

- Allow adequate rotation at the finish

- Help with balance as we post up.

Hugely Important! And yet, most recreational golfers perform no proper core exercises whatsoever. Not unless they are my clients. Luckily, you have now become my client by caring enough about your health and your golf game to take the advice in this book.

What Your Assessment Says About Your Core

During your self assessment, several exercises and drills evaluated your core strength and the ability for your core to stabilize the body. The muscles we primarily focused on are the upper back muscles, the anterior core (the abdominal musculature) the gluteal and hip muscles, and the low back muscles, including the visible external muscles, as well as the inner spinal muscles called the multifidi. But, remember, everything on the body is attached, and a weak core shows up in many different ways in many different tests.

The Overhead Squat Test is a whole body core assessment. A perfect squat with arms over head, requires strong upper back muscles, anterior core muscles, glutes and spinal muscles. Often, unless significant flexibility issues are a culprit, one may fail the squat test *because* of a weak core. If you could not perform the overhead squat test, but have normal flexibility, I would recommend:

-Abdominal strengthening such as planks, side planks, physio ball rollouts, standing anti-rotation exercises, and other plank variations. The consistent variable here is training the muscles of the spine to hold the spine *still* under duress. (Other more advanced core training techniques will involve rotation with speed such as medicine ball throws, but we still must always begin with working the spine through stability first)

-Gluteal and hip strengthening exercises such as bridges, dead lifts, lunges, hip abduction and squats. Yes! To get better at squats…. practice squatting.

- Upper back strengthening (the upper back is part of the core too- it holds shoulders back and down and stabilizes the upper spine) such as rows, pull-ups, planks.

The Bridge Test specifically tested the strength of the gluteals- the buttocks muscles- often called the "king" of the golf swing. If you had trouble with the bridge, either cramping in the hamstrings or wobbliness and shaking, you need to improve the strength of your glutes. Recommended exercises are: supine bridges, two legs or one leg, hip thrusters, dead lifts of all variations, lunges and squats.

The Single Leg Balancing Test looks at the stability and strength of the core as well as the hip muscles. Poor balance is often more related to core instability than ankle instability. Exercises recommended are: glute strengthening, lateral hip strengthening such as clamshells or lateral walking, bowler's squats. Practicing balancing on one leg is also a great way to "fire up" the core muscles so they learn to contract and stabilize the body during unstable movements.

The Torso/Hip Rotation Test gives us information about the anterior core as well as whether you can rotate the upper body and the hips separately. If you have the flexibility to rotate these body parts, but can't seem to keep one part still while rotating the other, then this could be a sign of a weak core. Strengthening the abdominals (there are several to work on) will help.

Ideally, you should perform these exercises every other day, beginning with 1 or 2 sets, and then work up to 3 sets to challenge yourself further. Planks and other isometric exercises should be held 15 seconds up to 30 or 45 seconds. No need to hold any longer! If you can hold for longer than 45 seconds, it's time to increase the difficulty of the exercise, not hold longer. Other exercises can be performed for 8-10 reps each. You can choose up to 3 exercises per area worked, but even 1 exercise can make a huge difference in core strength over time.

It's important that you tune in with *where* you feel the exercise. Abdominal exercises should be felt primarily in the abdomen, with only mild sensation in the back muscles. Glute exercises and hip exercises should also be felt specifically in those areas. If you do have more pain or discomfort in an area *other* than the muscles you are working, stop and check in, as this may mean you are doing the exercise improperly, or that you are overly fatigued.

The exercises shown below and on the following pages are by no means a complete list. But, these are the most doable and user friendly. The exercises are in ascending order of difficulty, in other words, the first exercise in each list is the easiest, and exercises get progressively harder. Most of the exercises shown below work multiple muscle groups at once. For example, anti rotation exercises work the glutes and abdominals. Note that some exercises will be found in the next chapter, which covers whole body strength training in more detail.

Spinal Stabilization Exercises

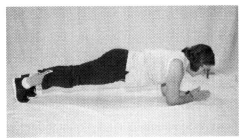

Plank -

PLANK- Works the anterior core, glutes and back muscles. Make sure elbows are directly under shoulders at start. Lift up from floor with abs engaged, glutes tight. Feet hip width apart. Hold for 10-30 seconds depending on strength.

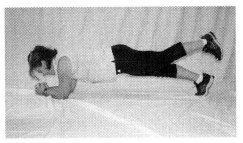

Plank - One Leg Lifted

PLANK WITH 1 FOOT LIFTED- Advanced version of plank. Lift 1 leg slightly off floor. Do not allow hips to drop or rotate. Brace abs and squeeze glutes for core stability. Hold for 10-15 seconds, then switch legs.

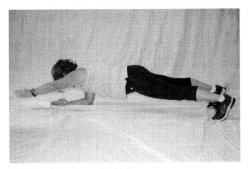

Plank - One Arm Lifted

PLANK WITH 1 ARM LIFTED- Advanced version of plank. Make sure you can execute regular plank before trying this. Lift 1 arm slightly off floor, then other arm, alternating for 15- 30 seconds. Do not lift, drop or rotate hips. Keep feet wide.

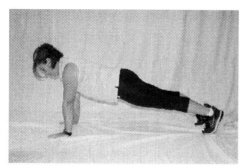

Push Up - Start

PUSH-UP START- The ultimate core exercise. Form must be perfect. Engage abs and glutes at start of exercise- body straight as a plank.

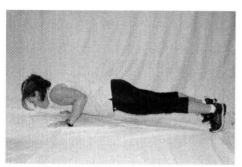

Push Up - Bottom

PUSH-UP BOTTOM- As you lower chest towards floor, squeeze shoulder blades together, keeping elbows from splaying to sides. Can be done on elevated surface to make it easier.

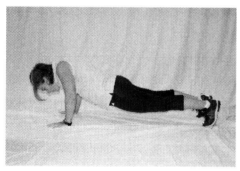

Push Up - Bad Form

PUSH-UP BAD FORM- Note here that my head has dropped, as have my hips. This indicates a weak core and bad form. If this looks like your push-up- elevate hands on couch or bench.

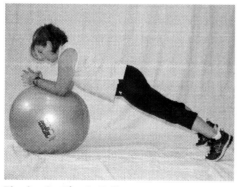

Plank - On Physio Ball

PLANK ON PHYSIO BALL- An advanced version of plank. If you can do traditional plank for 30 seconds with ease, try it on the physio ball. Feet can be slightly apart. Make small circles with elbows for a greater challenge. Form must be perfect.

PHYSIO BALL FOREARM ROLLOUT-
Start by kneeling behind the ball in neutral spine, abs tight, glutes engaged, back perfectly straight. Keep this form throughout exercise.

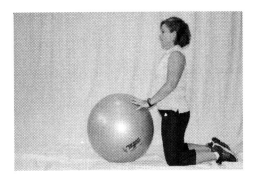

Physio Ball Forearm Rollout

PHYSIO BALL FOREARM ROLLOUT
Roll out on ball on forearms. Elbows can be bent or straight- but make sure entire spine remains still, abs tight, glutes tight. Pull back to start using arms, but with attention to keeping body rigid.

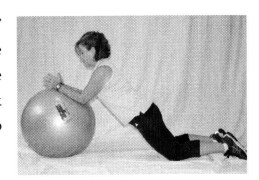

Forearm Rollout - Mid

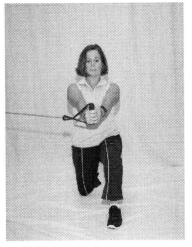

Half Kneel Palloff Press

HALF KNEEL PALLOFF PRESS- This anti-rotation exercise is ideal for golf. It can be done in a half kneel position, or full kneel. In half kneel, push hip forward of kneeling knee and engage abs. Arms are straight at chest height.

HALF KNEEL SIDE VIEW- Note tall posture, chin in neutral. Hold position for 10-30 seconds on each side.

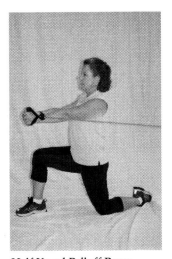

Half Kneel Palloff Press

Buttocks And Hip Strengthening

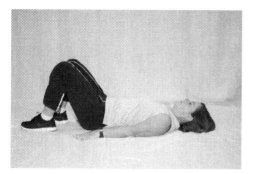

Two Leg Supine Bridge - Start

TWO LEG SUPINE BRIDGE- Lie on back with spine in neutral. Head and neck relaxed. Engage glutes and lift hips up into the air, pressing through the heels, squeezing glutes.

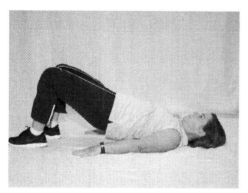

Two Leg Supine Bridge - Mid

TWO LEG BRIDGE- Do not over arch through low back. Lift is from the glutes and core, not the back or knees.

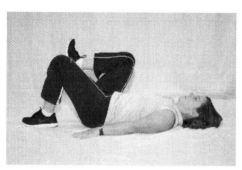

Single Leg Bridge

SINGLE LEG BRIDGE- Once 2 leg bridge is easy, single leg bridge is next progression. Bring one knee into chest and keep it there. Push hips up into air using heel of foot on the floor.

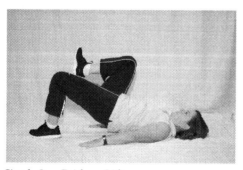

Single Leg Bridge - Lift

SINGLE LEG BRIDGE- Exercise should be felt in the glutes and hamstrings, primarily the glutes. Do not use low back muscles.

BIRD DOG- Begin on all fours, knees under hips, hands under shoulders. Engage abdominals and carefully lift one arm and opposite leg. Low back must remain perfectly still. Can be done alternating arms only, or legs only, as easier variation.

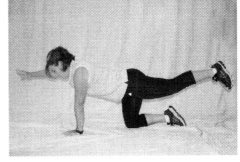

Bird Dog

CLAMSHELLS- Lie on side with knees bent and forward of body. Keep back totally still as you open up (abduct) hip. Feet stay together as you squeeze lateral hip and glute muscles. You may use a band for additional difficulty.

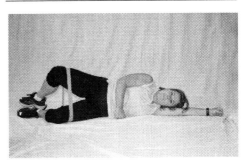

Clamshell Band

BOWLER'S SQUATS- Works lateral hip muscles as well as entire core. Great for balance and knee health. Reach with same arm as leg that is lifted. Bend ankle, knee and hip of stationary leg as you reach. Back must stay straight.

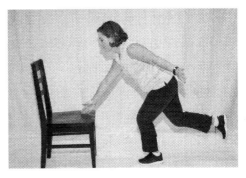

Bowler's Squats

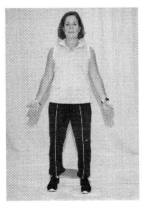

Lateral Walk - Start

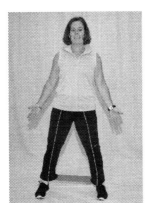

Lateral Walk - Mid

LATERAL WALK WITH BAND- Place band around ankles and stand with good posture, tension on the elastic band. Step sideways with a bent knee, using lateral hip muscles. Keep upper body still and back straight.

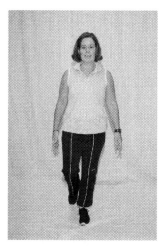

Standing Leg Balance

SINGLE LEG BALANCING- Practicing balancing on one leg is great for golf and great for challenging core stability. Keep aware of glutes, hips and abdominals as you balance. They should be engaged and working.

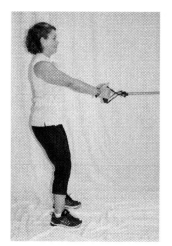

Standing Row - Start

Upper Back Strengthening

STANDING ROW- Stand with knees bent, abs engaged, one handle in each hand. Chin in neutral. Stand back far enough to have tension on elastic tubing.

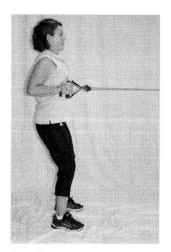

Standing Row - Mid

STANDING ROW- With thumbs up, pull handles into side of chest, squeezing shoulder blades together and keeping shoulders down. Release slowly back to start.

ONE ARM ROW- Place both handles in one hand for more resistance. Using shoulder blade area of upper back, pull handle next to chest. Squeeze shoulder blade towards spine but keep shoulder itself down.

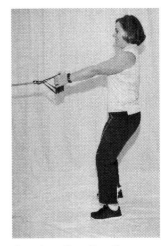

One Arm Standing Row

TWO ARM ROW ON ONE LEG- For a fun variation, try a two arm row standing on one leg. Combines balance work with core stability work.

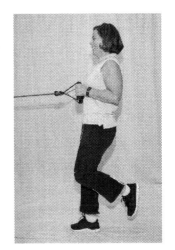

Two Arm Row One Leg

BENT OVER DUMBBELL ROW START- A bent over row requires greater core awareness, and teaches you how to keep good upper body posture during the golf swing. There are many variations of this exercise. Always keep the spine straight, shoulders down.

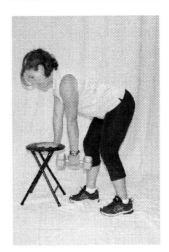

Dumb-bell Row Start

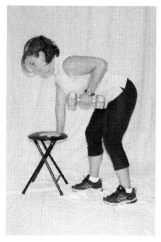

Dumbbell Row - Mid

BENT OVER DUMBBELL ROW- Pull dumbbell up into ribcage using lats and upper back, keep shoulder itself down and squeeze shoulder blade towards spine. Back must remain perfectly straight.

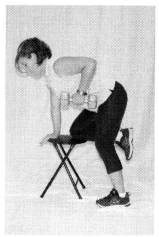
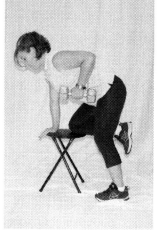

Kneel Dumbbell Row

KNEEL DUMBBELL ROW- VARIATION Placing the knee on the bench as you row gives you more support. One hand, or no support, is a more challenging variation. Always keep back straight with no rounding.

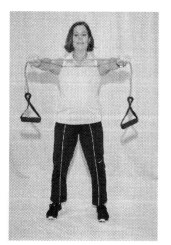

Brady Band - Start

Brady Band Series For The Upper Back

BRADY BAND START- For upper back endurance and good posture, try the Brady Band Series. Use light tubing held straight out at chest height. Thumbs point in. All movements return to this starting point.

SHOULDER ABDUCTION- With elbows still, but slightly bent, pull handles out using back of the shoulder and mid back. Squeeze shoulder blades together. With control, return to start position.

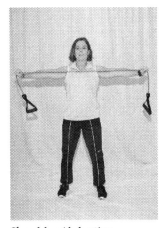

Shoulder Abduction

DIAGONAL SHOULDER ABDUCTION- Next, abduct arms with one arm pulling on diagonal upward, other arm pulling diagonal downward. Keep shoulders down throughout exercise and do not use elbows to create movement. Return to start position.

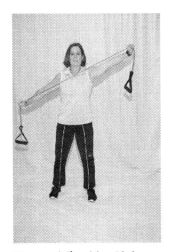

Diagonal Shoulder Abd.

DIAGONAL SHOULDER ABDUCTION- Repeat in opposite direction, noting any assymetry in strength. Return to start.

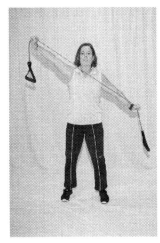

Diagonal Shoulder Abd.

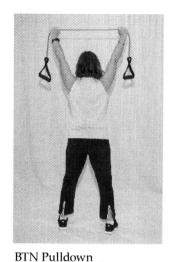

BEHIND THE NECK PULLDOWN- For last part of Brady Band Series, bring arms up over head with tension on elastic, palms face forward. If you can not bring arms directly over head, skip this part of series.

BTN Pulldown

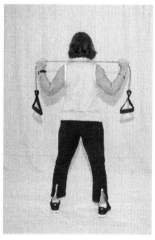

BEHIND THE NECK PULLDOWN- Keeping tension on tubing, pull elbows down into back of ribcage, squeezing shoulder blades together and down. Keep chin in neutral-do not jut chin forward. Do not pull tubing outward with elbows.

BTN Pulldown - Bottom

Chapter 6 - Whole Body Strength

As we discussed in the previous chapter, strength training has come a long way since the days of Arnold Schwarznegger and bodybuilding. Proper strength training programs work the body as a whole, just as nature designed. Unless you are training for a sport that requires a specific body part to be super strong, (like arm wrestling!), your strength training program should be comprised primarily of exercises that work multiple muscle groups at once. The exercises we covered in Chapter 5 fulfill this requirement. For some of you, you may choose to perform just the exercises from Chapter 5, and that's fine. They are very beneficial to your health and your golf game. But, for those of you who want more work, or are looking to change your body composition , the exercises discussed in this chapter will be necessary to add in to your programming. If you choose to do so, you will combine the exercise you chose from Chapter 5 with the exercise you choose from this chapter to form a whole body workout that you perform 2-3 times a week. This will take 45 minutes to one hour to perform, so make sure that you have a schedule that can accommodate this increased work load. At the end of the book, I will give you sample whole body workouts to choose from, as order of exercises and exercise selection is crucial to a safe, effective program.

Finally, two questions which may be circulating subconsciously in your brain need to be answered:

Will I lose flexibility from whole body strength training?

It's the elephant in the room......the myth that is most likely to be believed by recreational golfers. The final answer is... NO..... as long as you include flexibility work in your exercise regimen. In fact, recent studies published in *The Journal of Strength and Conditioning Research* [1,2] demonstrated that a proper strength training program executed correctly improved flexibility just as much as a stretching program. Now, I would not recommend strength training as a way to enhance flexibility, but this study is interesting and assuring. You can be BOTH strong and flexible, the perfect combination for golf.

As a woman, will I get muscles that are too big and bulky?

This is the most common question my female clients ask when I tell them they need to do strength training. As I have mentioned in previous chapters, unless you are genetically gifted and lift extremely heavy weights with the perfect nutrition to support muscle growth, NO, you will not. Most women just do not have enough testosterone to bulk up. And "bulking up" is a choice, not an accident. You would have to make a concerted effort to add enough muscle so that it changes the way you look for the worse. Most women look better from strength training, not worse. One caveat- some women do experience a circumferential body size increase from strength training. This only occurs when the woman is training very heavy, but eating excessively at the same time. You can increase the size of your muscles without losing the body fat over them if you do not watch your nutrition.

In Chapter 5 , I mentioned the tests that evaluated strength, and suggested exercises to address any strength deficits. This chapter includes a more complete list of exercises that are traditionally used to improve strength, an essential aspect of living a healthy life and having a great golf game. As before, these are listed in ascending order of difficulty. Choose the exercise that best matches your current fitness level.

[1] *Influence of Moderately Intense Strength Training on Flexibility in Sedentary Women*, Santos et al, Journal of Strength and Conditioning Research, 24(11):3144-3149, Nov. 2010

[2] *Resistance Training vs. Static Stretching: Effects on Flexibility and Strength*, Morton et al, Journal of Strength and Conditioning Research, 25(12):3391-3398, Dec. 2011

Some trial and error may be necessary, but always defer to the easiest exercise when beginning.

The major areas we need to strengthen in a whole body strength training routine are:

Anterior core- the abdominals

Upper and mid back

Legs- thighs, hips and glutes

Chest

Shoulders- rotator cuff

Each workout should include exercises for each of these areas. Choose 1 or 2 exercises per area and repeat that exercise for 1-3 sets, depending on baseline fitness level, for 8-15 reps. No need to do more than 15 reps of any exercise. If you can, it is too easy. If you cannot complete 8 reps, it is too hard. Do less work if you are just starting out. Push yourself more if you are an experienced exerciser.

DO expect delayed onset muscle soreness or, DOMS. This means that, 24-48 hours after training, you may experience mild to moderate muscles soreness. This is normal. Joint pain or intense muscle pain is not normal. Seek medical attention if this occurs. If injury or excessive soreness occurs, rest and ice are the best for all musculoskeletal injuries until you see your doctor. But, if you start slowly, pay attention to your form and posture and don't try and do too much too soon, this won't happen! And, luckily, as you perform the routine more frequently and you begin to get stronger and more coordinated, soreness will lessen anyway. This is not a sign that the program is no longer working. If you are working hard during the strength training session, then it is working. There is no advantage to being sore after every workout, so lessening of DOMS is a good thing!

Lastly, don't forget to always warm-up before hand and stretch after. This will improve your workout, reduce risk of injury, and lessen soreness. Well worth the 10 minutes.

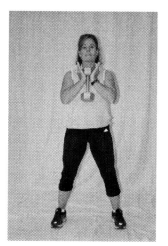

Goblet Squat - Start

Hip And Leg Strengthening

GOBLET SQUAT START- With feet hip width apart or slightly wider, toes pointed straight ahead or slightly out, hold 1 weight on chest with chest up, good posture, head in neutral.

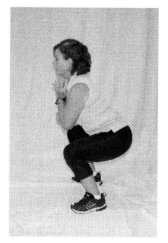

Goblet Squat - Side

GOBLET SQUAT SIDE- Sit hips back into heels, keeping spine upright with no forward rounding. Ideally hips should drop at or below knees. At bottom of squat, begin to exhale and press up to start.

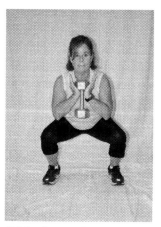

Goblet Squat - Front

GOBLET SQUAT FRONT- Keep weight evenly on both feet, chin in neutral. Do not let knees cave in, nor jut out.

HAMSTRING PULL-IN START- Lie on back with feet on apex of ball. Relax head, shoulders and neck.

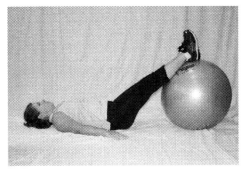

Ham Pull - Start

BALL BRIDGE- Using glutes and hamstrings, lift hips into air into a bridge.

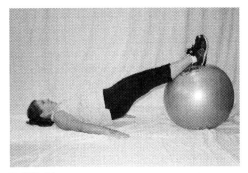

Ball Bridge

HAMSTRING PULL-IN- Keeping hips up into air, pull ball into buttocks using heels. Use arms to stabilize if necessary, but do not put pressure into neck. Return to start with control.

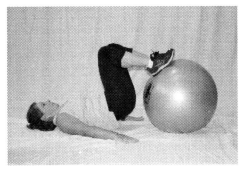

Ham Pull - Mid

HAMSTRING PULL-IN SINGLE LEG VARIATION- When 2 leg pull-ins become easy, try it with one leg, with the other leg up in air and stationary. Much more difficult.

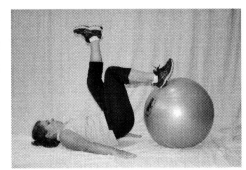

Single Ham Pull

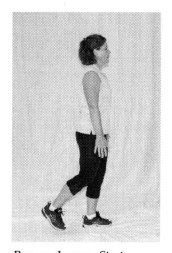

Reverse Lunge - Start

REVERSE LUNGE START- Reverse lunges are great for working glutes and hips, and for balance as well. Start with tall posture, chest up, knees soft.

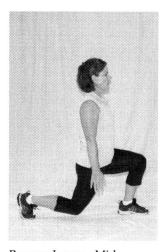

Reverse Lunge - Mid

REVERSE LUNGE- Step back, lowering knee towards floor in a wide stance with knees at right angle. Keep spine tall, then press back to start with heel of front foot. You should feel this in the glutes and hips of stationary leg.

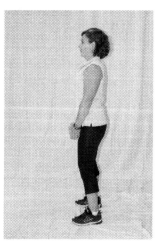

Dead Lift - Start

DEAD LIFT START- A dead dift is great to work glutes and hamstrings and to help with posture. Always start with perfect posture and maintain this throughout entire exercise. In this variation, hold one weight in front of hips. Feet hip width apart.

DEAD LIFT MID- Lower weight slowly down body, hingeing at hips as you sit hips back, weight into heels. Back stays perfectly straight. Keep chin in neutral, shoulders back and down.

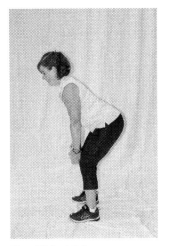

Dead lift - Mid

DEAD LIFT LOW- Continue to lower weight down close to body with slight bend in knees, (but keeping knees still). Only go as far as you can until you feel stretch in hamstrings. Squeeze buttocks and hinge back up to start.

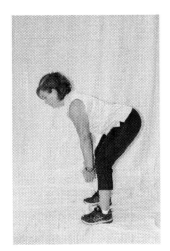

Dead lift - Low

SINGLE LEG DEAD LIFT START- A much more challenging version is a single leg dead lift. You may hold one weight in each hand, or just one weight on same side as leg that will lift back. If using one weight, hold other arm out to side for balance.

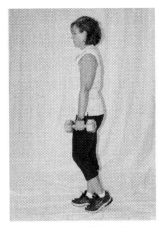

Single Leg Dead Lift - Start

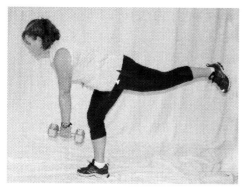

Single Leg Dead Lift

SINGLE LEG DEAD LIFT- Keep weights hanging close to your body- hip hinge, lifting one leg behind as weight lowers. Keep entire spine straight or slightly arched- no rounding of any part of the back. At bottom, engage glutes, and "scissor" back up to start, using glutes and hamstrings, not low back.

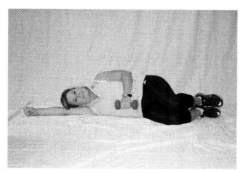

Side Lying - Start

Rotator Cuff Strengthening

SIDE LYING EXTERNAL ROTATION- There are many ways to strengthen the rotator cuff. This exercise is quite safe and golf specific. Lie on your side with a very light weight in your hand, palm down, upper arm into side.

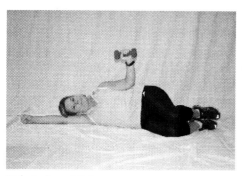

Side Lying - Mid

SIDE LYING EXTERNAL ROTATION- With upper arm glued into side, rotate weight up, keeping wrist in neutral (Put a small pillow under arm if you have any pain in front of the shoulder). Work should be felt along back of arm and shoulder.

Chapter 7- Improving Balance

Most of us don't think about balance until we lose it. Whether you are standing on a ladder, walking on uneven surfaces, stepping on ice, or addressing the ball on a downhill lie, balance is something that should just be "natural". Unfortunately, it often feels like work. Many of my clients get concerned about balance after they experience a fall or slip, only then realizing that their ability to keep their balance has diminished. This is related to multiple factors that affect our balance in a negative way; age, sedentary lifestyle, disease and injury, poor flexibility and a weak core, not to mention inner ear problems, which are very common. Luckily, we can control many of the factors that affect balance with exercise!

Aside from disease, balance is really a combination of strength, flexibility, proprioception and adaptation, in other words, practice. (Proprioception is the complex neuromuscular process that gives our body feedback about movement and spatial orientation. Proprioceptor organs are located throughout the body in the tendons, but also in the inner ear. Proprioception can be improved through balance work.)

Physically, balance is not related to one particular joint, like the ankle, as many people believe. In fact, it is more related to our center....our core.... and how well we can maintain a stable center of gravity. Sure, ankles and feet play a big role in good balance, but it is a culmination of many physical factors which allow us to stabilize our joints on varying surfaces. We can train balance like any other physical attribute. And we do it with multiple types of exercise- strength, flexibility, core , proprioception, and practice!

Unfortunately, golf has a way of highlighting poor balance, although you may not always recognize it as such. If you have difficulty on uneven lies, if you hang back on your finish, if your putting is off, this could all be related to balance. What makes golf even more unfair is that, for an important part of the game, we are standing still…at address…in static posture, preparing to swing the club. In our address, our body is forward, bent from the hips. We need to be able to hold this static posture with a proper spine angle, and even more importantly, hold this spine angle during our swing. Of course poor balance will affect your set-up, and without a well balanced set-up, well…you know what happens to your swing.

One other thing to mention; balance diminishes with age. Our eye sight, vestibular system, neurologic systems and proprioception are all affected as we get older. Diseases common in seniors such as deafness, vision problems, arthritis, diabetes and Parkinson's Disease have a huge impact on balance as well. So if you are a "senior" golfer, you may want to create a fitness program that emphasizes exercises that help with balance.

During your golf fitness assessment, you were asked to balance on one foot for as long as you can. How long did you last? Professional golfers can stand on one leg for over 20 seconds with their eyes closed. Closing the eyes takes away vision, which is one of the senses that help us with balance. I did not ask you to do this because I find most people have difficulty enough with their eyes open! So, if you had a lot of difficulty with the single leg balance test, this is your chapter! Once you get better at single leg balancing and single leg exercises, you can retest yourself. See if you improve your time, and even try the test with your eyes closed.

Many of the exercises we have discussed in previous chapters address balance as well as other aspects of fitness. There is a crossover impact on balance from most components of fitness. These exercises are listed below with the chapters in which they can be found.

Bird Dog- Chapter 5

Elastic walking and other hip exercises- Chapter 5 and 6

Bowler's Squats- Chapter 5

All abdominal exercises- Chapter 5

Bridges- Chapter 5

Lunges- Chapter 6

Dead Lifts- Chapter 6

I also recommend exercises that involve actual single leg balancing techniques such as Bowler's Squats, vector reaching, balancing on an uneven surface such as a disc or core board, and single leg variations of traditional exercises and yoga. You can choose one or two exercises that challenge your balance and incorporate these into your workout regimen. Some of these exercises are shown below and on the following pages:

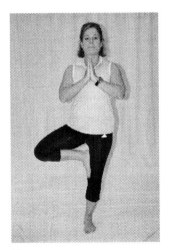

Tree

TREE POSE- This yoga pose is challenging both mentally and physically, and is great for balance. Engage glutes of standing leg as you calm your mind and body. If you begin to lose balance, return foot to floor and rest.

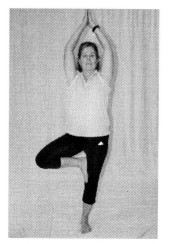

Tree with Arms

TREE POSE VARIATION- For a greater challenge of balance, raise arms over head, keeping shoulders down and space between ears and shoulders. Make sure you are breathing steadily through out exercise to calm the mind, just as in golf!

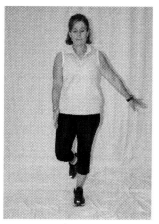

Vector Reach - Start

VECTOR REACH START- A more challenging variation of Bowler's Squats, this exercise asks you to reach to the ground while standing on one foot, bending at your ankle, knee and hip, but not your back.

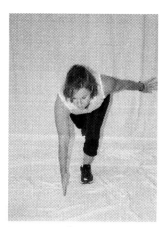

Vector Reach - Front View

VECTOR REACH FRONT VIEW- Reach to the floor at various positions to challenge balance and core stability. Keep knee of standing leg centered on foot, not diving in or dropping out.

VECTOR REACH SIDE VIEW- Note similarity of position to Bowler's Squats. Reach to points on the floor as on a clock- noon, 1pm, 2pm 3pm, 11am, 10am, 9am.

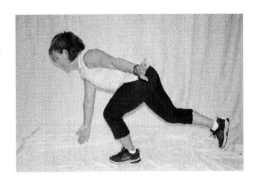

Vector Reach - Side View

WARRIOR YOGA POSE- Builds balance, core stability and body awareness. Shoulders are relaxed yet strong, thighs working in lunge position. Heel of front foot aligns with arch of back foot. Do not lean forward, keep spine over hips.

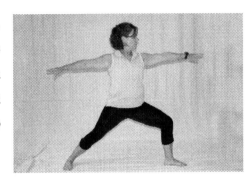

Warrior

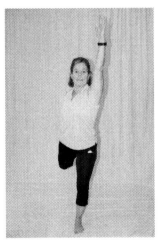

Dancer - Front

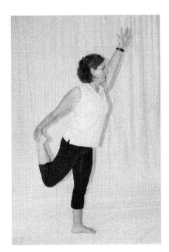

Dancer - Side

DANCER'S POSE- This challenging pose requires flexible thighs and chest muscles as they counter stretch each other. Pull heel into buttocks lengthening thigh muscle. Reach straight arm up and slightly forward, but do not over arch back.

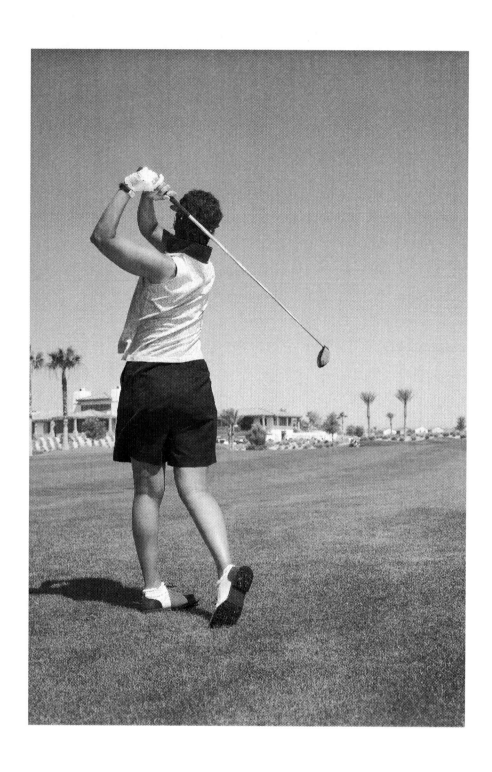

Chapter 8 - Golf Warm-ups and Cool-downs

Imagine Annika Sorenstam rushing up to the course at the LPGA Championship, grabbing her clubs out of the trunk of her car, running over to the first tee, and hitting her first drive. A ridiculous thought, isn't it? And yet, this is what most golfers think is a normal pre- game ritual for golf. I never understood this norm. Coming from the fitness industry, warm-ups and cool-downs have been ingrained in my brain, and for good reason. So essential are these practices, that every professional athlete performs a whole body warm-up routine and post exercise stretching. If every professional golfer warms up prior to a match, and cools down after, why shouldn't we?

Warm-ups for exercise or sports are essential to consistent performance and reduction of injury and post exercise soreness. It prepares the body both physically and mentally. Warm-ups should mimic the movements of the specific sport, allowing the body and brain to "groove" the neuromuscular patterns that define the sport. In today's strength and conditioning world, warm-ups consist of dynamic stretches- flexibility through movement (as we have discussed in previous chapters) - followed by a period of light sports demands. For example, the professional golfer may warm-up dynamically, do some light stretching with a trainer, and then head to the range to practice. They follow a very specific routine that relaxes them mentally and physically. This is something all golfers, no matter what the skill, should be doing.

Unfortunately, most amateur golfers either do not warm-up at all, or perform warm-ups that do not facilitate neuromuscular activation. The average warm-up I see on the course is the type of warm-up that may actually decrease power in your swing! This is because most amateur golfers perform static stretching before golf, stretching that quiets the neuromuscular system instead of activating it. As mentioned in previous chapters, prolonged, intense static stretching, prior to the golf game, has been shown to decrease distance and power output. This decrease in strength does not just apply to golfers. It is standard practice in sports to warm-up with dynamic stretches rather than static. So, if you have not been warming up, or do not know what type of warm-up is best for you, it's time to change this up and learn the latest techniques for proper sports and exercise warm-ups.

Cool-downs are also very important for injury prevention and to decrease delayed onset muscle soreness. Cool-downs encourage muscles and other soft tissue to relax and heal. Post exercise is the best time to stretch for elongated periods. Sports and, exercise in general, are repetitive activities that stress soft tissue. Over time, without post exercise stretching (or proper warm-ups), chronic pain and injury can result. If you have ever felt stiffness and pain after a golf game, whether it is the same day, or the next, then you could benefit from a good cool-down.

Warm-ups

Your warm-up should be dynamic in nature, but should also address your individual physical needs. If you are typically tight through the hips, emphasize loosening them up in your warm-up. If your shoulders and chest are tight from computer or desk work, make sure you spend extra time improving their flexibility. If you need more of a mental prep, take more time to swing the club at the range. The best warm-up is a combination of both.

Shown below are several warm-up exercises, stretches and preparatory movements that address the areas most commonly in need of help. I always recommend that you begin your warm-up with self myofascial release techniques using either the

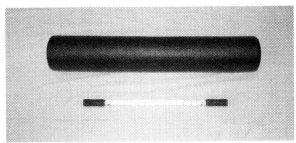

foam roller or one of the more portable tools like "The Stick" or a "Tiger Tail". These tools can be purchased easily online at any sports performance website. They are not readily available in most sporting goods stores. You'll note that the first few exercises are

Self Myofascial Release Tools- Foam Roller and "Stick"

standing and dynamic. I like standing stretches for golf because...you guessed it... we stand for golf! Plus, most golfers can't lie down on the first tee to stretch. Not appropriate. However, I did include Cat and Cow yoga poses which you can do in the privacy of the locker room if you'd like.

Perform dynamic movements 10-15 x each. Remember that these movements should be gentle at first so as not to strain anything. Once you get the tissue warmed up, if you have a few problematic areas of tightness, go ahead and statically stretch these, but only briefly. Hold these static stretches 5-8 seconds and repeat 2-3x per area. Static stretches are listed below as well.

Dynamic Warm-ups (See chapter 4)

Cat and Cow

Standing Knee to Chest

Standing Leg Swings

Standing or Sitting Cross
    Leg Hip Stretch

Arm Swings

Torso and Hip Rotations

Static Stretches (See chapter 4)

Kneeling Hip Flexor Stretch

Hamstring Stretch

Chest Stretch

Lat Stretch- with club

Shoulder Stretches- with
    and without club

Cool-downs

Unlike cardiovascularly demanding sports like soccer or basketball where a cool-down that includes light cardio activity is necessary, the cool-downs I recommend for golf are static stretches only. Golf is very repetitive, but is also a sport of true "power", where maximal effort is often used during the golf swing. Muscles and their attachments get pretty cranky after this type of activity. Static stretches, where the stretch is held for 30 seconds or more, relaxes the stressed muscles. (Post golf is also a great time to get a massage, but if you can't, try foam rolling and then stretching) Never bounce or force these stretches. Take the stretch to where you feel the light "stretch pain", and then breathe. Deep breathing while statically stretching signals the muscle to relax even more. It is best to repeat the stretches 2-3 x each. Listed below are some basic stretches that are great for after golf. Some are the same as the warm up stretches above; the only difference is the length of time you hold the stretch. Short for the warm-up, long for the cool-down. (See Chapter 4 for photos of stretches.)

Cat and Cow- still dynamic

Side Lying Twist (yoga)

Hamstring stretch- lying or standing

Cross legged hip stretch- seated or lying

Quadriceps/hip flexor stretch- standing or side lying

Calf/achilles stretch-

Chest stretch

Lat stretch

Shoulder stretch

9

Nutrition and Hydration

Hopefully, *"Getting Golf Ready"* has given you a great overview of how to improve your golf game, as well as your health and fitness. Flexibility, core strength, whole body strength and balance, are all integral parts of a healthy body and a healthy golf game. As Tara Parker-Pope discusses in her column "What Your Golf Swing Says About Your Overall Health", posted in the *NY Times,*

> *"While golfers often focus on improving their swing and lowering their scores, sports medicine researchers and golf industry experts increasingly are focusing on the links between golf and health. They are finding that everything from the quality of your swing, to the yards you get from your drive can provide telling insights into your overall fitness and health."*

Wow. She says it all! And to think, you are ahead of the game already because you cared enough about your golf game and your health to buy "Getting Golf Ready." So, congratulations are due. However, optimal health and golf performance are contingent not only on physical preparation, but also on your nutrition and hydration practices. In other words, what you put into your body determines what you put out! Well fueled, well hydrated muscles work better. And good nutrition and hydration, with adequate vitamins and minerals, helps muscles, tendons and ligaments tolerate the exercise stress that can lead to injuries.

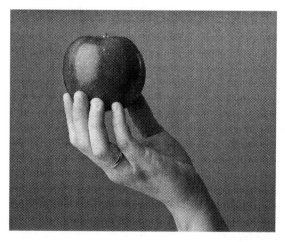

Perhaps you have never considered that what you eat and drink before, during and after your golf game impacts your golf performance. But it certainly does. I think we often forget that golf is a sport….a long sport. A sport that takes anywhere from 3.5- 5.5 hours to play. Can you think of any other sport- recreational or otherwise- that takes this long to play? Your golf game can encompass two meals of time and you may burn up to 1000 calories during a golf game depending on your skill, the course, and whether you carry, pull or ride. And, moreover, in the heat and humidity, dehydration is a big risk as well.

Poor nutrition- poor fueling and poor hydration- can turn a good golfer into a crummy one. Muscle fatigue and subsequent loss of power and strength, not to mention loss of mental focus, are all immediate issues associated with poor nutrition and hydration. Have you ever noticed how your performance and energy diminishes late in your golf game? I would venture to say that almost all of us have noted low energy and overall fatigue during a round of golf. Of course this is related to skill and overall health, but nutrition and hydration are of equal importance. Now, if your goal is just to get outside, have fun and get some sunshine, you may not need to care too much about your golf nutrition. But, if you are more serious about your game, if you desire to improve your score and feel as good on the 18th hole as the first hole, then, nutritional diligence is a must for you.

Daily Nutrition

Good nutrition is a day- to-day battle. We often allow our "nutrition" to get too complicated, too worrisome. I think there are some basic rules we can all adhere to that encompass good nutrition, without getting too neurotic and worried about it. Listed below are my Top 10 Tips For Good Nutrition.

Top 10 Tips for Good Nutrition

1. Drink water throughout the day. Dehydration is a major cause of low energy levels and sabotages sports performance as well as weight loss efforts.

2. Know how much is in a "portion" of the foods you eat. Many of us eat two or three portions of our foods without knowing it. A portion of pasta is the same size as a scoop of ice cream. A serving size of juice is 6oz, not 12oz.

3. Include protein, carbohydrates and healthy fats at every meal and every snack. Your body needs these fuels consistently dispensed through the day.

4. Eat every 4 hours to keep energy levels high and blood sugar levels constant. We actually burn calories when we eat, and small frequent meals expend more energy than one or two meals a day.

5. Eat the majority of your calories during the day, when you will burn them up, rather than at dinner time when they are more likely to get stored as fat.

6. Keep sugary foods and starchy carbohydrates to a minimum. Most nutrition professionals agree that these are the foods which are the main cause of the obesity epidemic we are now facing.

7. Avoid excessive alcohol consumption. Drinking too much alcohol will sabotage your efforts to maintain a healthy weight, as your body stores most of it as fat. Alcohol also lowers your resolve to eat healthy! Furthermore, alcohol is a depressant and is dehydrating, so it should not be a fluid of choice for the golf game.

8. Choose healthy, whole foods that are as natural as possible. Fruits, vegetables, lean meats, healthy fats and high fiber whole grains are all a necessity. Avoid processed foods, fast foods and prepackaged foods as they contain unhealthy fats and high levels of sugar, salt and chemicals. (The healthiest fats include those found in avacados, olives and olive oil, some seed and nut oils, and the oils from fish)

9. Take a whole food supplement and an Omega-3 Fatty Acid supplement. As a

woman, you may need to take a calcium supplement. Consult with your MD. You may also need to take a Vitamin D supplement as well, as many of us have inadequate Vitamin D levels. As far as a whole food supplement, there are many, but I personally recommend Juice Plus+, a whole food alternative to vitamins. It is the most natural way to get the necessary vitamins, minerals and phytochemicals our bodies need.

10. Eat breakfast whenever possible. Those who skip breakfast risk a slowing of metabolism and low energy. Research has shown that those who skip breakfast always end up eating more later in the day anyway! Your breakfast is truly the most important meal of the day. Go high in protein, whole foods and healthy fats, and low in sugars and processed foods. Eggs, high protein cereals, protein smoothies, yogurt, nuts, fruit and whole grains are all great breakfast foods.

Pre- Game and Golf Nutrition

When it comes specifically to golf, eating within 1-2 hours of your game is advised. Using the rules above, choose a healthy pre-round meal that includes lots of protein, healthy carbohydrates and good fats.

Next, take some time to prepare a snack, or another meal, for the course. While some golfers eat along the course, perhaps at the turn, choices at the "grille" are often poor. Hot dogs, chips, soda? Not good for sports performance. Would you eat these foods during your gym workout? I doubt it. And, high fat foods, like those served at the turn, can cause immediate negative physiological consequences by slowing down blood flow to the heart and other organs. From a general health standpoint, this is a bit scary. Add in dehydration and multiple full strength golf swings, and you do have a recipe for disaster.

Good snacks for the course follow the same basic rules. A sandwich with protein on 100% whole grain bread, fruit and nuts, a yogurt with fruit, some crackers and cheese, a healthy protein bar, even high protein cereal mixed with dried fruit and nuts can be a great "on the course" treat. Avoid high sugar snacks. While sugar is a quick "pick me up," it is also an equally quick "put me down", as blood sugar drops very quickly with sugary snacks. This will definitely impact your energy levels within a very short period of time.

Hydration for Your Golf Game

Proper hydration is so key for mental clarity and physical performance that it can not be taken for granted. How much fluid to take in depends on your resting state of hydration, your exertion level, length of the golf game,

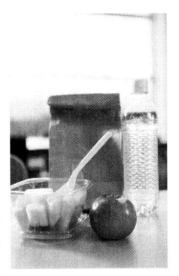

and the weather, specifically heat and humidity. This is the biggest factor that contributes to dehydration and possible serious complications of heat illnesses. Cold weather can also impact hydration, so don't be fooled when golfing on a cold day, but let's face it, most of us golf in warm and humid conditions where we are sweating out much needed body fluids. In general, drink plenty of water before, during and after golf. 32 oz. or more may be necessary over the course of the round.

Because the golf game can last so long, sports drinks are appropriate in some cases. However, I always recommend that you cut sports drinks in half with water, as they often are a bit too sugary for good health. Sports drinks are no miracle. Personally, I just drink water and have a piece of fruit, and this has the same positive affect. However, sports drinks are a quick way of getting some electrolytes and water in your system as fast as possible. They can be especially helpful in situations where you already are feeling poorly from dehydration. But, let's not wait to get there. The truth is that if you are feeling thirsty and tired, you are already dehydrated. Get some fluids in your body quickly!

For overall health, more and more scientific research is proving that proper hydration is crucial to weight maintenance and weight loss. Dehydration can cause feelings of hunger, so, often, we may reach for food when, in reality, we are just dehydrated. When you are feeling hungry, but not sure if the hunger is real or timely, have a nice cool glass of water first. See if this takes care of the hunger. Adequate hydration also keeps the metabolism humming. Dehydration slows down the metabolism.

One area of controversy is the amount of water we should be taking in each day. Most of us have heard the mantra of 8-10 glasses of water a day. I think this is generally great advice. But if you are the type of person who has trouble drinking this much water, take heart. Many nutrition experts believe that the fluids from fruit and vegetables as well as other liquids, are equally as important as plain old water when it comes to hydration.

Making Nutritional Changes Stick

When it comes to improving your nutrition and hydration, just like improving your golf fitness, small steps make a big difference. Start with incorporating one or two new nutritional habits into your lifestyle. Once you are successful with these new habits, move forward by adding more improvements. Keeping a food log is a helpful way to track these new habits. I often recommend that my clients keep a detailed food log which tracks specifics of every meal, portions of foods, times of meals and snacks, as well as fluids taken in. Keep a log for at least a week, and if you have aspirations for weight loss, even longer. Those individuals who keep a food log are 60-70% more likely to lose weight than those who do not keep a log.

If you have difficulty with the time and details of a food log, I have also included a **Nutrition Checklist** for you. You can also tailor it for you individual needs by changing any one column to help you achieve a specific goal.

The good news is that any positive changes you make are one step closer to better health. Good health means a happy life and a better golf game!

Getting Golf Ready • **Nutrition Checklist** • **Week:**

Item	M	T	W	Th	F	S	Su
8 Glasses H2O							
2-3 Fruits							
3-5 Veggies							
Protein at every meal							
Healthy Snacks (list)							
Junk Food" (list)							
Ate every 4 hours							
Took vitamins/ supplements							
Ate when hungry							
Did not get "overfull"							
Exercise Or fun play (list)							
Slept 8 hours							

NOTES:

Getting Golf Ready • Golf Fitness Assessment Worksheet • Week:

Test	Pass	Fail	N.I.*	Notes:
Postural Assessment	☐	☐	☐	
Pelvic Tilt	☐	☐	☐	
Overhead Squat	☐	☐	☐	
Ankle Dorsiflexion	☐	☐	☐	
Single Leg Balance	☐	☐	☐	
Torso Rotation	☐	☐	☐	
Hip Rotation	☐	☐	☐	
Lat Flexibility	☐	☐	☐	
Shoulder Flex Test 1	☐	☐	☐	

*N.I. = Needs Improvement

Test	Pass	Fail	N.I.*	Notes:
Shoulder Flex Test 2	☐	☐	☐	
External Rotation	☐	☐	☐	
Buttocks Strength	☐	☐	☐	
Hamstring Flexibility	☐	☐	☐	
Quad Flexibility	☐	☐	☐	
Hip Flexor Flexibility	☐	☐	☐	

*N.I. = Needs Improvement

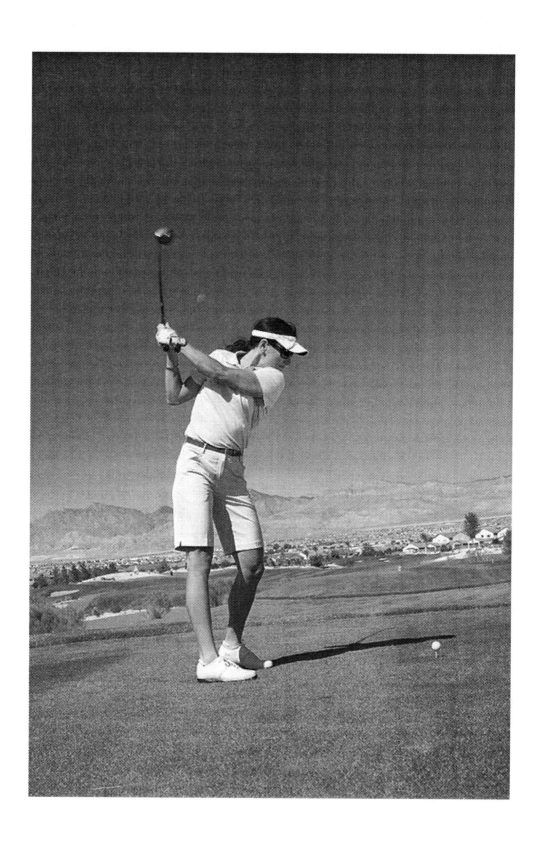

10

Your *Getting Golf Ready* Sample Golf Fitness Programs

The programs suggested are sample programs, giving you an idea of how I generally structure a workout. You may use these exact programs, or substitute other exercises from Getting Golf Ready as desired. Make sure you speak with your physician before beginning this or any new exercise program. You may have a medical concern that may impact your ability to perform these exercises, and so your doctor must be consulted.

You'll note that there are exercises to strengthen the whole body as well as target golf muscles. Flexibility is addressed both before and after the workout. However, depending on the results of your golf fitness assessment, you may want to add additional exercises to address any weaknesses or flexibility issues.

The programs shown are in two phases- the first- Phase 1- for more novice fitness enthusiasts, and the second- Phase 2- for intermediate fitness levels. The program should be done 2x/week minimum, with 3x/week even better, as long as you have plenty of rest between workouts. Often, you may need 2 days between workouts if you are sore, so do take that time if necessary.

Always warm-up before your exercise session with foam rolling or stick rolling, paying special attention to the areas that are tight or painful, as they need extra work. Next, perform brief stretches, 5-10 seconds, and repeat each brief stretch 2-3x. Do as many dynamic warm-ups as possible pre-exercise.

You can circuit exercises with no rest in between to save time and keep you moving. Pair up two or three exercises and alternate them. For example, once warm-ups are finished, do 1 set of the first 3 exercises in a row with no rest, repeating this mini circuit 2-3 times. 2 sets of each exercise may be enough in the initial few weeks, but after 2-3 weeks, you should try and perform 3 sets of every exercise (which would be 3 runs through the mini circuit).

Always stretch after your workout, especially your tight or problem areas. Post exercise, static stretching is best, and stretches can be held 30 seconds or longer if desired.

Do expect mild to moderate "delayed onset muscle soreness", more moderate if exercise is new for you. However, delayed onset muscle soreness- DOMS- does not mean joint pain, only soreness in the muscles themselves. If you experience any unusual joint pain, or muscle pain that lasts longer than a couple days, consult your physician.

Golf Fitness Program for Getting Golf Ready- Phase 1

Exercise	W/R/S	Notes	Record dates exercise/program is perform							
Foam roll or stick roll whole body	20x/area	Especially side of thighs, low back								
Kneeling Hip Flexor Stretch	3x/side	Hold briefly -8-10 secs each								
Cat and Cow	10x									
Seated Torso Turns	5x/side	Add No Money if shoulders tight								
Leg Swings	10x each way	Front and back and side to side								
Supine Bridge- 1 or 2 legs	3 sets of 10	8 reps if single leg								
Planks on forearms	3 sets of 15-30 secs									
2 Arm Standing Row with tubing	3 sets of 12									
Reverse Lunges	3 sets of 8x/leg	Add weights when easy								
Push-ups- can be elevated	3 sets of 6-8	Hold abs in, butt tight								
Single Arm Row w/tubing or Dumbbell Row	3 sets of 10/arm	Dumbbell row uses free weights								
Lateral Band Walking	2 sets of 8x each way									
Side Lying Shoulder External Rotation	2 sets 8x/arm 3-5 lbs	Always start with low weight								
Restretch: cross leg stretch	Hold 30 secs each									
quadriceps, hamstrings, chest	Hold 30 secs each									

Exercise	W/R/S	Notes	Record dates exercise/program is performed									
Foam roll or stick roll whole body	20x/area	Especially side of thighs, low back										
Kneeling Hip Flexor Stretch	3x/side	Hold 5-10 secs										
Lie on roller lengthwise	10x	" No Money" shoulder warm-up on roller										
Lying Side Twist	5x/side	Opens up chest and shoulders										
Windshield Wipers	10x											
Single Leg Bridges	3 sets of 8x/ leg											
Side Planks	3 sets 20-30s/side											
Pull-ups or Inverted Rows	3 sets of 5-8	Inverted row can be done on barbell in squat rack										
Reverse Lunge/Single Leg Dead Lift	3 sets of 6	Combination exercise- do 1 of each 6x/side=12 reps										
Push-ups	3 sets of 10	Lift 1 leg if easy For ½ reps										
Single Arm Kneeling Dumb-bell Row	3 sets of 8x/arm	Go heavy										
Lateral Band Walking	2 sets of 8x/each											
Brady Band Series	2 sets	1 set is 4 reps of each movement										
Restretch: cross leg stretch	30 secs											
quads, groin hamstrings, calves, chest	Hold 30 secs each											

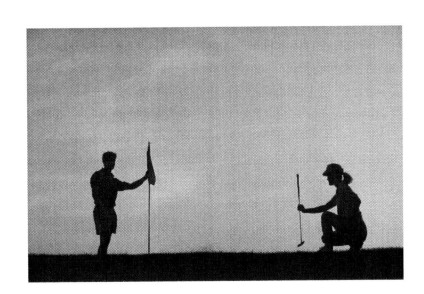

Getting Golf Ready
Yoga for Golfers

by Kathy Ekdahl

Yoga and golf; a match made in heaven, right? Maybe. Maybe not. It seems intuitive—yoga promotes flexibility and golfers need flexibility. Yoga promotes balance and core strength, and golfers need balance and core strength. And, the mind body piece of yoga can be a huge contributor to the mental quietness that golf often demands. But, where do you start? What kind of yoga is right for you and your body, and your body's specific needs? Most importantly, what yoga poses could hurt you or be too risky for your body?

If you are an experienced yogi or yogini, these yoga questions may already be answered, but even you could benefit from a greater understanding of the yoga poses that would most improve the golf swing and your *individual body*, and that's what we hope to do for you!

A Brief Introduction to Yoga and its Parts and Principles

For those of you unfamiliar with the history of yoga, yoga is an ancient tradition that dates back more than 4000 years. One of the world's oldest know written texts, the Rig-Veda, contains elements of yoga as practiced by Hindu priests in India. Although yoga was created in ancient India, its timeless principles of honoring the strength and power of the human body, while simultaneously emphasizing inner awareness, self- focus and meditation, make it perfectly suited for today's busy lifestyles.

Yoga is neither a sport nor a religion. It is a journey of the body and mind, where the union of the two nurtures your life energy, or, as it is called in Sanskrit, your *prana*. Yogis believe that our health is dependent on the free flow of *prana*, (sometimes called chi) in our body, mind and spirit. Eastern philosophy believes that the mind and body are used as a vehicle for the expression of the spirit. When the spirit realizes its true potential, (through, for example, a yoga practice) it transcends mind and body resulting, finally, in "enlightenment."

In yogic thought, the body contains seven energy centers called *chakras* (wheels). The *chakras* store *prana* and correspond to and control various parts of the physical and spiritual body. In order to achieve true enlightenment, all of the *chakras* must be awakened, thus allowing *prana* to be released up the spine, reaching "Nirvana".

Hatha Yoga, (considered the "mother" of all forms of yoga),as well as most other types of yoga, joins the body, mind and soul in the path to enlightenment by awakening the *chakras* through a series of postures called *asanas*, breathing exercises called *pranayama*, and meditation. The postures used during yoga class vary greatly from easy sitting postures, to difficult balance or strength poses. In our western thought processes, we may think certain poses are more special or more important because they are difficult or advanced. But in the eastern mind, all yoga poses, regardless of difficulty, are equally essential. This is important for westerners to remember as this is what makes yoga so great. No matter what your skill level, you will succeed at your yoga practice because yoga always honors the individual. Yoga is not about ego or competition! Although your body will get strong and flexible through yoga practice, the physical changes are only important because the physical body holds the most important part of us, our spirit.

Yoga in the New Millennium

I truly believe yoga can be for every body, at every age. It develops core strength, flexibility, posture, balance, energy and focus. Yoga is about "living in the moment", being present and comfortably aware of every breath, every muscle, every thought. It has been scientifically proven that yoga improves and restores health and well-being and reduces chronic stress. Yoga has been shown by research to improve flexibility much better than other traditional forms of stretching because the poses are held longer with more attention to posture and detail. Many poses and postures are even now used in traditional western exercise and physical therapy. Almost all of the traditional strength exercises and mobility and movement prep exercises "us" personal trainers recommend come from yoga. All lunges, squats, planks, bridges, side planks, dead lifts, airplanes, hip flexor and hamstring stretches, supermans, quadruped, push-ups, thoracic spine mobilizations, piriformis stretches, are variations of Yoga poses. So, we need to give credit where credit is due.

So, whether you seek more traditional enlightenment and quietness of the mind, or are merely interested in getting stronger, more flexible and improving your balance, yoga is here to stay. And, it can be a great addition to any existing exercise program or sports regimen.

Now, to be picky, many of the types of yoga we practice nowadays have been greatly westernized...and this is both a good and bad thing. Good, because westernized yoga is more appealing to our culture of exercise and fitness. Good because millions of people have tried yoga in their local gym, senior fitness class or yoga studio. The more the merrier. But, westernized yoga has its negatives too. When yoga was first introduced to the west, it maintained many of its safe, simple principles. But like everything in this millennium, things are moving faster than ever and yoga has changed dramatically from its origins. Yoga has become the "workout fad" of the decade. The yogis of past would be horrified! Along with Pilates, it is touted as a "miracle" workout, guaranteed to lean you out, zone you out and promote all kinds of strength, while enhancing flexibility enough to make a pretzel jealous. Many types of yoga move along very quickly, matching our western attitudes, and can often become a competitive class, where yogis and yoginis try and outdo each other with fancy poses. This was not the original intent of yoga. Ancient Yogis, traditionally trained yogis, spend years- decades!- learning proper yoga postures and breathing techniques.... unlike us westerners, who want everything done fast and furious.

As fitness trainers and coaches know, this westernization of yoga can also be unsafe. And, safety is a major concern for me as a trainer, coach and yoga instructor. In fact, many trainers avoid yoga completely, labeling it as a recipe for injury, and they are correct, to a large degree. Extreme postures such as headstands, shoulder stands or over-arching or over-rounding of the back, have been associated with significant injuries. Many yoga classes do not provide the correct type of stimulus for our golfing goals. They either contain all flexibility work, which can, in the long run, produce hypermobility and injury risk, or they move too fast, not allowing proper form and technique, which can increase the risk of injuries to golfers.

So, for golfers (and other athletes,) it has to be the RIGHT kind of yoga class, a yoga class that addresses the areas of tightness and weakness that are most common in golfers. But how does the average golfer (or trainer for that matter) know what type of yoga class is safe and helpful and what poses will increase injuries and create poor performance? This yoga overview will hopefully educate the golfer to what to look for in a yoga class, how to create your own yoga program, and, most importantly, what poses to avoid.

13

Yoga: The Good, The Bad and The Ugly - An overview of the benefits and risks for golfers

In an article I wrote for strengthcoach.com and several golfing websites including golfgurls.com, I overviewed my opinions on yoga for golfers. As a yoga instructor myself for over 17 years, I love yoga! But, education is key. Yoga, like any movement based regimen, has risks and benefits. And, as determined golfers, we need to reap the benefits without incurring the risks. Getting hurt in yoga, while trying to improve golf flexibility, just does not work for me, and I certainly don't want it to happen to you. Let's look at the benefits first.

The benefits:

Yoga is phenomenal for teaching proper breathing. Many of us (especially women who have been holding their stomachs in for decades!) do not breath properly- we either hold our breath during improper times or breathe from the upper chest, not the diaphragm and belly, where the deep anterior core muscles lie. Until we learn proper breathing, we will never be able to correctly activate some of the anterior core muscles, which are a key factor for back safety and club head speed and power during the golf swing. Breath awareness also leads to postural awareness and release of physical tension. Are you aware of where you hold tension? Are you aware of your unhealthy postural tendencies? Perhaps not. For golfers, carrying tension in the shoulders and neck, or addressing the ball with poor posture, has a significant negative impact on the golf swing. I have found that sitting quietly in a yoga class, focusing on breath, posture and awareness of physical tension or relaxation, can be of great help to golfers. Later, we will explore in more depth the Yogic "3 Part Breath", the foundation of all relaxation, meditation and awareness. It will be a huge help for you, the golfer, as you approach the first tee, or are getting ready to sink your putt for the club championship.

Another important benefit of yoga is that yoga teaches the golfer to stay present and focused even in times of physical, mental and emotional stress. Hold the pose Down Facing Dog for a few breaths, and you learn patience and presence in your body, even while feeling mildly uncomfortable. In yoga, we do not try to disconnect, but instead, connect to our feelings, physical as well as emotional, and then explore these feelings with patience and awareness. For golfers, it's easy to imagine the benefits of staying present and focused with each individual shot, rather than thinking about outcomes, or the last shot, or the next one...all recipies for disaster. Yoga can even teach patience as you wait in the line at the bank!

And, the most obvious benefit of yoga; yoga greatly enhances flexibility, balance, core stability and postural awareness- all key elements to a good golf game. For example, even our golf address can be enhanced by yoga as our address requires good core activation, a sense of proper balance and weight shift, and of course, great posture to create an optimal spine position. Many golfers cannot even achieve a proper address due to physical weaknesses and muscular tightness. If you cannot address the ball in an optimal position, you'll never have an optimal swing.

Now the risks —

The first year I taught, I followed a cookie cutter method of teaching yoga. I utilized poses that were traditional and common- like Uttanasana-forward bend with extreme lumbar flexion (rounding of the low back). My back was killing me! Duh! Since then, I have completely overhauled my class and taken out any and all poses that don't meet the standards I follow when training my clients. Coming from a fitness background helped me modify my class to be safe, and to target the physical areas of the body that most people need work on. Unfortunately, some yoga teachers do not fully understand kinesiology, biomechanics, back safety and injury prevention. They do not take a detailed medical history and thus are unaware of individual physical issues, which is essential. Some yoga poses may not be appropriate for EVERY body, as some poses can cause injury or aggravate existing conditions. For example, Cobra or Up Facing Dog is disastrous for students with some back conditions like spondylolethesis, or fractures of the spine. Sustained lumbar flexion as in a forward bend? Sciatica city. Yoga should never cause injury- only help heal injuries. So, coming from a fitness background will help me *help you* love yoga, while keeping injuries at bay.

One of the biggest issues I have with our westernization of yoga is that yoga has become sped up, heated up, competitive. This is the opposite of the traditional yoga mindset of no ego, quiet awareness and moving with proper form and execution. When deconditioned students join "Power Yoga" or "Hot Yoga", they frequently get injured. All new students should master slower, more precise forms of yoga before trying any of these faster/hotter classes. Yogis and yoginis (female yogis!) spend years learning just one pose. Yet we think we can learn and master 26 in one class? In addition to excessive speed and too many ego driven poses, some hot classes require taking class in 105 degree heat... yes 105 degrees. As most of us know, working out in heat can be very unhealthy. Yet, the hottest type of yoga- Bikram Yoga- is also one of the most popular because it has been marketed for weight loss and cleansing.

One last caveat —

Yoga is being marketed as "the everything" workout- just like Pilates, Zumba or other new exercise regimens. This does a great injustice to an ancient form of spiritual growth, exercise and discipline. Contrary to how yoga is currently marketed, the truth is that yoga does not make "lean long muscles", and most yoga classes do not create a large calorie deficit. Madonna and other yoga loving stars are not thin from yoga, but from eating celery and air for 10 years. Yoga is not a substitution for strength training, as it only builds strength with bodyweight and isometrics- clearly not enough for most of us who golf, play sports or do physical work. So, as much as I love yoga, it is just ONE part of a comprehensive golf fitness program that should also include strength specific to golf, consistent teaching from your golf pro, and a dedication to frequent practice.

Yoga has become popular enough that a large segment of our population is trying it out. Unfortunately, most yoga students are not educated enough to know what they should and should not do in class. Some students may need flexibility work while others need strength work. Unfortunately, yoga classes often focus on hypermobility- excessive flexibility- which new students may think is proper and necessary! And yet, excessive flexibility, or the attempt to achieve it, is the cause of many injuries. Golfers need flexibility AND strength to be the best they can be. As the old saying goes- "You can't push a wet noodle uphill" and for golfers… a wet noodle can't produce power during the golf swing.

Other cautions-

Many yoga classes do absolutely no warm up or movement prep. Imagine starting an exercise routine with a sustained forward bend?

This is very common in many forms of yoga. Proper movement prep and some static stretching are absolutely necessary before any faster more arduous poses are attempted. Getting Golf Ready Yoga will have you fully warmed up before you try any challenging poses.

There are many poses which, frankly, I feel are downright bad for everybody. Headstands/shoulder stands are really risky. Very few people have the scapular stability and neck strength to bear all their weight onto their head. I tried it once- competitive and compelled- and had severe neck pain for a week. Lesson learned! Other really nasty poses which can injure are Reclining Hero, Plow, The Wheel, Camel, Cobra (if not done properly, extreme backbends in general, free standing handstands (wall supported handstands are doable and fun! and all forms of lumbar flexion and twisting. I recommend that if you are new to yoga you skip some of these risky poses. Simple is best in the beginning.

So, remember, like all physical practices, yoga has its goods and bads. If we can learn to eliminate risky poses, and always include poses that address our weaknesses and build strength, yoga can be for every body. Yoga is a transformative practice. It connects the body and mind and teaches patience, contentment and body awareness- all things we hope to attain as a good golfer.

Now that you have a better understanding of what yoga can and cannot do for you, the golfer, let's explore in more detail the benefits of yoga, starting with proper breathing.

14

The Three Part Breath

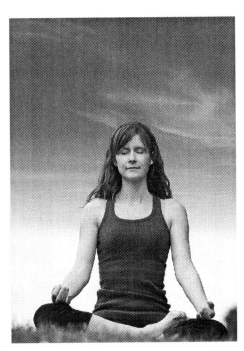

As discussed previously, yoga was primarily created as a way to relax the physical body, allowing for the mind to relax and let go of stress. A relaxed mind results in clarity of thought, solution solving space, and presence of mind. However, these qualities are not just for yogis! All of us negotiating the hurried, complex world we live in can benefit greatly from practicing a quiet mind. Athletes, in particular, have found that clarity of thought, positive mindset, and a relaxed demeanor during their sport is a key to long term success. Too much energy, too much aggression and too much overthought is the death of a natural athlete. Successful, natural athletes respond to the pressures of their sport with confidence and awareness. In my opinion, no sport requires more confidence, awareness and necessity to stay in the moment, than golf. Practicing yoga with its accompanying breath work allows us to "practice" what we need to bring to our busy lives and, for golfers, to our golf game.

Outlined on page 109 is the start of "practicing" how to quiet the mind. If your mind is busy-busy, please be patient with yourself. Remember that even one breath with true awareness is the start of something great! We all must start somewhere.

The type of breathing which is traditionally used in yoga is The Three Part Breath. In typical yoga classes, we begin the class with a few minutes of seated mediation and breath work, just as you can practice below. At the end of class, we also take time to find our breath again after the rigors of the poses (asanas). This part of class is called savasana, or "corpse pose" because we now lie on the floor to quiet the mind. It works. Students leave the practice feeling energized, calm and yet fully aware and present in the moment. Our deep breathing is not about sleeping or dreaming. It is about creating the conscious mind *you* want, an ancient tradition.

More recently, science has backed the essential nature of relaxing the mind. Dr. Herbert Benson, founding President of the Mind/Body Medical Institute at Harvard, conducted a study back in the early 1970's. This study showed that there is a direct *physiological* response within the body when it is in a relaxed and/or meditative state. This study resulted in the publication of a book called the *"Relaxation Response"*. Dr. Benson states "The relaxation response is a physical state of deep rest that changes the physical and emotional responses to stress... and is the opposite of the fight or flight response."

Dr. Benson suggested doing this process twice a day for 20 minutes. For those of you who have practiced meditation previously, please feel free to use whatever technique works for you. For those of you who have never meditated, we suggest starting smaller and build up. Even a few minutes of this practice will create a physiological response in your body, lessening stress and creating awareness.

The most important part of this exercise is to let go of any judgment at all. There is no right or wrong way. Do the best you can to be present and aware. You may find random thoughts popping in. This is perfectly normal. Just let them be and focus on your breath. Remember, all we are doing is bringing awareness to something we do unconsciously all the time.

- Sit with your feet on the ground and your back supported.

- Now, as you inhale, put your hands just below your navel and feel the air expand first into your belly , then into your rib cage, expanding the ribcage outward in all directions, and then finally and up to your clavicle. This is the Three Part Breath. Hold the breath there for a second.

- Now, very slowly release your breath, feeling the air leave your chest first, then your rib cage, then your belly.

- As you breathe say to yourself, inhale, exhale and keep repeating that. This will help you to stay focused on your breathing.

- Continue to breathe deeply and normally without forcing it, just feel the flow. Do it for as long as is comfortable.

- Don't over think this, don't judge how you're doing it, just play with it and practice it. This is important because when we take a full inhale we are filling our body with oxygen, feeding every cell, and when we exhale we release toxins. This is what Dr. Benson calls the relaxation response.

So, while deep breathing exercises may seem far away from the process of hitting out of a sand trap, it is not nearly as far as you think. Practicing deep breathing will create an awareness in both the body and the mind, allowing you to stay present with the task at hand. One of my biggest mental golfing mistakes is getting ahead of myself on the course, or ruminating about my last shot. This can be a disaster in a sand trap.

Proper breathing, using all our lung space, also allows us to also get in touch with where we hold our stress. For example, we may hold stress in the shoulders or neck or low back. This is often caused by improper, shallow breathing. We know that tightness in the upper body is a huge detriment to the golf swing, so, becoming aware of unhealthy postures through deep breathing can really help our swing. Moving forward, you can practice your breathing and postural awareness in the car, at work, waiting in line at the bank, or sitting in your golf cart.

15

Yoga Poses for Golf Warm-up

As a long time fitness professional, a warm-up is something I just take for granted. Whether it is for running, weight training or field sports, I *always* warm-up. Warm-ups, the right kind anyway, always reduce injury risk and improve performance. So, if this is a known... a given... for all sports, all physical activities, why don't golfers warm-up? Or should I say more specifically, why don't recreational golfers warm-up? ALL tour pros do! All professional athletes in all sports do! It's time you too step up your game and do the same.

In previous chapters of *Getting Golf Ready*, I discuss how to create a proper golf warm-up based on your individual body's needs. Hallmarks of a proper golf warm-up are dynamic, movement based mobility drills and some short static (no movement rather than dynamic) stretches to emphasize any extra tight areas you may have. So, yoga poses can be a great addition to any golf warm-up. Shown below are some of my favorite warm-up yoga poses. Some are simple, others more intense and complex. Choose what works for you.

You'll notice that these yoga poses primarily address hip flexibility, and there is good reason for this. Most golfers are pretty good at warming up the upper body, but not the lower. And yet, hip rotation and glute activation are the most important aspects of a proper golf swing! So- try these out (after foam rolling and dynamic warm-ups as covered in "Getting Golf Ready- An Introduction to Golf Fitness") for additional help for those tight hips.

Seated Cross Legged Hip Stretch: Great for pre golf or even during golf while in the golf cart. This pose stretches glutes and hip rotators and is a variation of lying cradle pose. Make sure spine is very tall, no forward rounding.

Kneeling Warrior: Also known as kneeling hip flexor stretch, one of my favorites. This pose lengthens front of hip and thigh to decrease back strain. Keep spine tall without arching back, push kneeling hip forward.

Runner's Lunge: A more intense version of a hip flexor stretch. Keep back as straight as possible, chest up, shoulders back and down, chin in neutral. Bend knee slightly on back leg to lengthen quadriceps more.

All 4's Groin Stretch: This is not a traditional yoga pose, but it is one of my favorite warm-ups which I do use in my yoga class. Get into all 4's, neutral spine or even "cow" spine (slight arch). Bring one leg out to the side, toe point forward, and sit back slightly until you feel a groin (adductor) stretch from pelvis to knee.

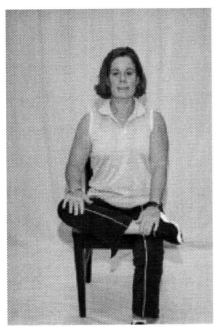

Seated Cross Legged Hip Stretch

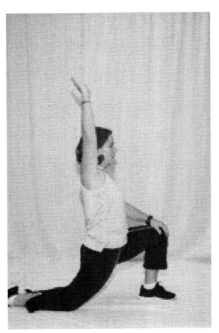

Kneeling Warrior

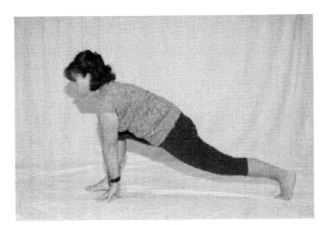

Runner's Lunge

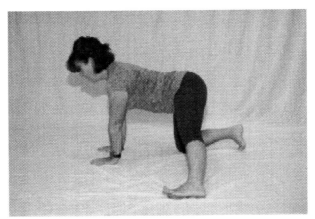

All 4's Groin Stretch

16

Yoga Poses for Golf Flexibility

As mentioned previously, yoga is best known for its ability to improve flexibility. Many golfers, mostly men, but also many older women, need significant flexibility help. What's important to understand is that the flexibility we need for a great golf swing comes from very specific places, and, so, your flexibility routine- aka stretching routine- needs to address these areas. Not only is it important to understand what body parts to stretch, we also need to realize that when one body part is stretching, other parts of the body are stabilizing, or holding still. This is why flexibility *and* strength go hand in hand. Without stabilization of some areas of the body via strength, your body would just contort and twist with every stretch. This is why yoga is such a useful tool for all forms of fitness improvement. In yoga, we both strengthen and stabilize with almost every pose, a perfect balance of work and rest, strengthen and stretch, yin and yan!

When practicing yoga for golf flexibility, the areas we primarily need to address are:
- Stretching the chest and front of the shoulders to obtain a more erect upper back during address, and to improve our shoulder turn.

- Stretching the upper back via thoracic rotation (twists) *while* the hips stay still, *and* stretching the hip muscles, especially the hip rotators, *while* keeping the upper back still. This separation of upper and lower body twisting is crucial to the golf swing. Yoga is perfect for this.

- Lengthening the hamstring muscles, located along the back of the thighs, which attach to the pelvis. More commonly an issue for men, women who sit for work can also have overly shortened hamstrings.

- Stretching the front of the thighs (quadriceps) and hip flexors (the muscles that attach thighs to front of hips) so that excessive strain is not put onto the back and so the abdominals can work properly.

- Keeping the lumbar spine mobile in both flexion (slight rounding) and extension (slight arching), as the golf swing necessitates both movements. What the golf swing should <u>not</u> do, is *cause twisting at the low back... ONLY at the hips and at the upper back. Attempting to twist the low back (lumbar spine) during your golf swing will cause injury. Doing the same during yoga is equally as bad.* For golf, the low back does *not* need to twist.

Here is a broad sampling of the kinds of yoga poses which are great for improving golf flexibility during your daily, or bi-weekly stretching/yoga regimen. You may also want to use these in your warm-up prior to golf, but these are, in general, a bit more complex, so they may be better suited for a separate routine. I particularly like the Cat and Cow and Standing Quadriceps stretch as warm-ups for golf. Please make sure you are well warmed up prior to these more complex poses. They should not be rushed. Stop immediately if you have any unusual pain or feel the pose is too intense. Create a short routine with the poses you most need, keeping a balanced routine to address all of the areas of golf flexibility outlined above. Yoga poses (asanas) that are joined together in one routine create a "yoga flow" or vinyasa. Repeat the vinyasa flow 3 or 4 times, and you'll notice that you are getting more flexible with each round. Congratulations! Now you are a real "yogini".

Lastly, many of these poses, and the poses shown in the warm-up chapter, can be done in isolation throughout the day to address tightness and stiffness from sitting or working at your computer. Keeping stiffness at bay with small bouts of yoga and stretching can also greatly reduce chronic pain and poor posture from sitting.

Cat and Cow: A perfect start to any yoga routine, cat and cow move the spine safely through flexion and extension. The lumbar spine both rounds and arches during different aspects of the golf swing, so this is essential for a healthy back. When rounding into Cat, exhale and pull abs in, tuck buttocks under, let head relax and hang loosely. In Cow, inhale as shoulders press down the back and you arch back and lift hips. Do not over arch neck, keep chin in neutral.

Lying Side Twist: Lie on your back, bend knees into chest and have palms face up. Face up is very important. Gently roll knees to one side and allow the body to relax. Allow the shoulders to relax into the floor. If your shoulders are very tight, they may kink up and feel like they can't relax to the floor. If this happens, move arm down towards body and breathe.

Runner's Lunge with Twist: Start with runner's lunge, as in warm-up. Twist first towards the front knee and raise arm up into the air. For a harder twist, twist away from front knee. Place back knee on ground for better stability.

Hamstring Stretch with Tie: I often do this early in my yoga class and at the end as well. If your hamstrings are tight, start with one knee bent on the floor. Ease slowly into the stretch, exhale and allow the hamstring to release.

If you are flexible, straighten the other leg on the floor. Press that leg down to enhance stretch. You can also try the Groin Stretch with the Tie, by pressing one leg down into floor, and slowly lowering straight leg to one side, holding the tie in one hand.

Standing Quadriceps Stretch with Club/Dancer's Pose: Note the similarity of these poses. Using your golf club for balance, you can do the first stretch on or off the course. For a greater challenge, work to the full Dancer's Pose, using 1 arm in air for balance, reaching up to sky, and pulling non standing leg slightly back, without overarching back. Make sure standing leg is strong and still, foot full to the floor.

Pyramid with a Twist: Pyramid is a wonderful pose for lengthening hamstrings and groin (adductor) but it is essential your back be completely straight. If you cannot get your hands to the ground and keep a straight back, place hands on a yoga block or stool. Keep toes straight ahead throughout. Be most careful getting in and coming out of pose. Feel free to go down to knees. Twist to both sides, palms facing away ONLY as long as low back is straight. This is an example of mid back twisting (as in the golf swing), not low back.

~ ~ ~ ~

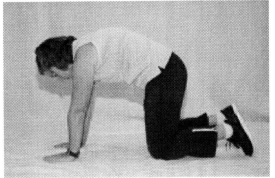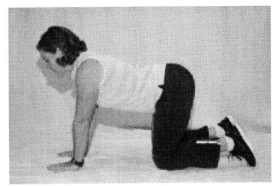

Cat and Cow

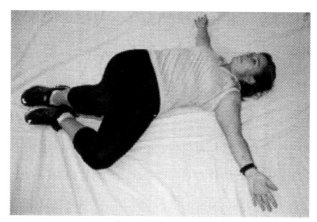

Lying Side Twist

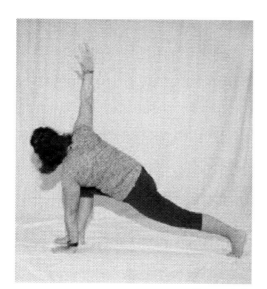 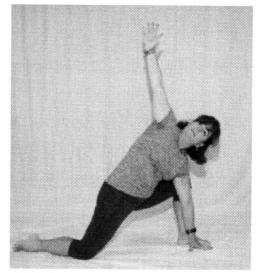

Runner's Lunge with Twists

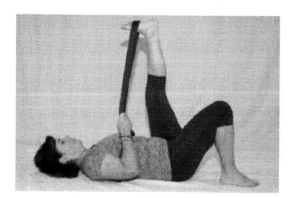 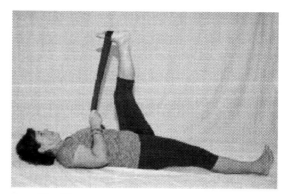

Hamstring Lengthening with a Tie

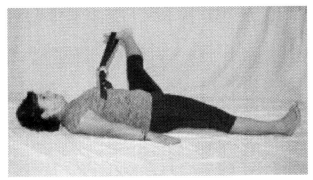

Lying Groin Stretch with Tie

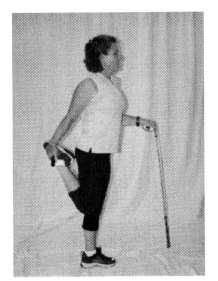 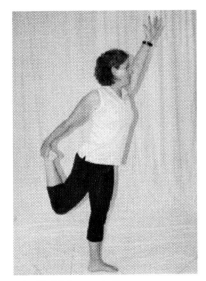

Standing Quadriceps Stretch with Club/Dancer's Pose

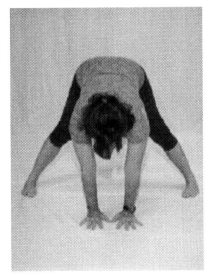 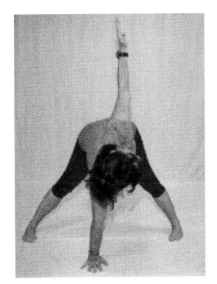

Pyramid with Twist

17

Yoga Poses for Strength and Balance

4000 years ago, Yogis practiced yoga for both spiritual and physical health. There are many yoga poses which are wonderful for core strength and stability and that strengthen the muscles of the body with "isometric" strength, strength in one stationary position. So, it is clear yoga can enhance some kinds of strength, but not all kinds of strength, and specifically not the power we know we need for good club head speed in the golf swing. I always advise all my clients to do conventional strength and power work to improve their golf game, and not to rely on yoga to do it all, because it cannot do everything! But, yoga can be a wonderful addition to any exercise regimen for variety and muscle endurance, and these positives will certainly help your golf game. I think the best use for yoga, from a fitness perspective, is for core endurance and stability. And, since core endurance and stability are what creates good balance and good posture on and off the course, you will notice I have also included balancing poses in this chapter. Good core stability= good balance. Balance is not merely a factor of what goes on at the ankles and feet, it is more about the hips and core.

Choose some or all of these poses to enhance your golf posture, balance and golf address. They can be done very day, or every other day with your strength routine.

Tree Pose: This is one of my favorite poses for calming the mind. The most challenging part of any balancing pose is the mind judging when you cannot do it well. Let go of judgment. Feel free to hold on to the wall to get into the pose, or for assistance the entire time. The raised foot can be placed in the upper thigh, or on the mid calf, but not on the inside of the knee itself. Stand tall and tight, chest up, breathing steady. Do both legs of course. Notice if you have one side better than the other? This may correspond to your swing faults.

Warrior 2: This is just one version of warrior pose and is great for building endurance in the shoulders and legs. Keys to this pose are: shoulders staying down, not lifted, spine erect, lunge deep with front foot facing forward, back foot angled slightly forward as well. Look forward over front arm as well.

Standing Cradle Balance: This is more difficult than tree pose. Feel free to hold onto wall and hold just one arm at the chest. Cross one leg over the other while standing, and sit your hips back, squatting slowly, keeping chest facing forward, not down to the floor. Do not let spine bend forward.

Warrior 3: Also called airplane, this is very similar to a single leg dead lift. The standing leg is strong and straight and the only bend in this pose is from the hip space, not the spine. Reaching towards a wall as a point of reference is a great way to get into this pose. You can also hold gently onto the wall or a railing for the duration of the pose.

Side Plank Variation: on knees and straight legs – While side plank is a standard strength exercise, it really comes from yoga initially. Side planks strengthen the shoulders and lateral abdominals as well as glutes and low back. Side plank on feet with straight legs is very challenging, so feel free to begin with knees and lower leg on the floor. Keep elbow directly under shoulder, then hike hips up in the air, keep hips way up., don't let anything sag.

Bridges: A traditional strength exercise as well as a yoga pose. In yoga, students often overarch the spine, but I do not advise that. Just keep spine in neutral if possible, and press hips way up into air. Keep buttocks tight.

Bird Dog: This pose works the core, and specifically the small muscles inbetween the vertebra, called the multifidi. It is also a great place to start to work on balance. Begin on all fours, and then, keeping attention to low back, slowly lift 1 arm and opposite leg. Draw abs in slightly to keep low back perfectly still.

Down Facing Dog: This pose is great for many aspects of the golf game. It lengthens hamstrings, calves and lats (mid back and lateral back muscles) and strengthens shoulders and upper back. Breathe – exhale- as you move from all fours, pressing hips back into the air and letting head and shoulders rest between arms Locked knees are not necessary nor optimal. Relax!

~ ~ ~ ~

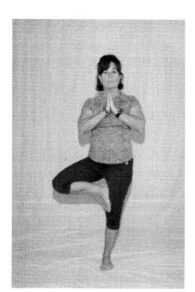

Tree Pose

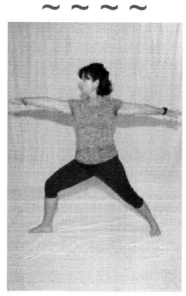

Warrior 2

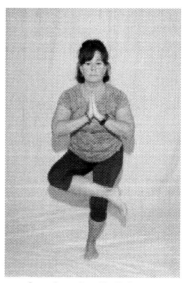

Standing Cradle Balance

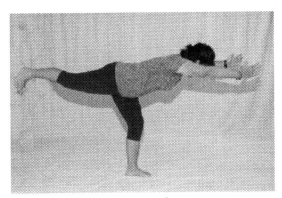

Warrior 3

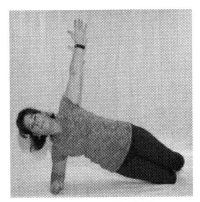 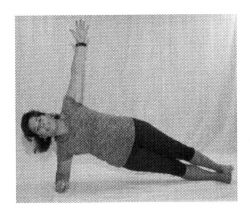

Side Plank Variation - knees and straight legs

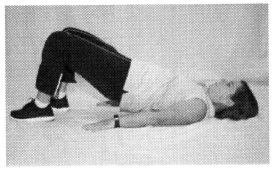 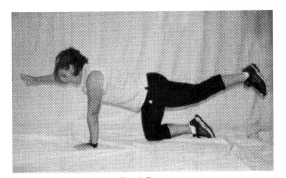

Bridges   Bird Dog

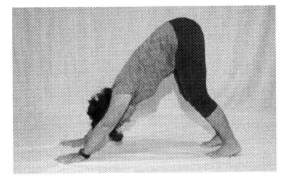

Down Facing Dog

In Conclusion...

I grew up in a family of golfers... that is, if you were male! My brothers and father golfed weekly, but I was never invited. It was probably for the best at that time. They would usually come home from a game of golf arguing with each other. My brother would've thrown his clubs several times over the round, or my father would have spent most of the round "correcting" my brother's golf game. Neither was conducive to a relaxing afternoon and neither sounded like fun.

But, at age 42, after changing jobs and having extra time on my hands, I took up golf myself. It was hysterical at first. I clearly remember the first time I went to the driving range. It must've taken me over 60 balls before I hit one good shot. I was thrilled and must've looked it, because just then, I heard a lone clap behind me. Another golfer had been watching my pathetic attempts to hit the ball and clapped after my one and only good shot. What a funny story that guy had to tell. I can only imagine how poor my swing mechanics were back then. Now, 10 years later, golf has turned out to be one of my favorite things to do. I find golf challenging, fun, enjoyable and relaxing. The beauty and quiet of the golf course are things I truly enjoy, even if my score is not always what I hope for. And, while I may not be able to run or lift heavy weights when I hit my 70's and 80's, I know that I will be golfing!

Getting Golf Ready comes after years of working on my own game, which has progressed relatively well, mostly due to good coaching by my golf pro, but, of equal importance, my good health and fitness. My golf game is certainly not great, but I continue to improve. There is no question in my mind that good fitness is essential for good golf. And, while there may be some unfit golfers who score well, their potential for improvement is low, and their potential for injury, high. I'm looking for the opposite potential and, I hope you are too!

Getting Golf Ready is by no means the only good guide to golf fitness. There are many great books filled with golf fitness exercises and drills. My goal is a bit different. It is not to merely give you golf exercises, but to help you understand the "why" of golf fitness. It is to show you that the same exercises which help your golf game will also improve your fitness, decrease your chronic pain and help you feel stronger in your day-to-day life.

No golf fitness instruction would be complete without mentioning the essential role of the golf pro. *Getting Golf Ready* is not meant to teach you how to swing a golf club, and in my personal training practice, I never give my clients advice in that manner. That is the job of the golf professional. I highly recommend you check in periodically with your golf pro. I am always so amazed when I hear amateur golfers say that their golf pro "messes up their swing" and hence their game. That's ridiculous. That's a sign that a golfer has poor swing mechanics, and just does not want to do the work to improve them. Golf is not the kind of sport you can play without occasional feedback from your pro, or without consistent practice and diligent work off the golf course.

If you have any ideas for golf fitness you'd be interested in learning about, please contact me at kathy@personalbestpersonaltraining.com Or, if you have any specific questions about your own golf fitness, feel free to email me as well.

For more information about Getting Golf Ready visit these websites:
http://www.golfgurls.com
http://www.personalbestpersonaltraining.com

Biography

Kathy Ekdahl, BA, CSCS, is a nationally certified personal trainer and strength and conditioning coach with over 28 years experience in health and fitness, including working for a decade as a gym owner. She is a TPI Certified Golf Fitness Instructor and brings years of experience as a yoga teacher to help golfers reduce their risk of injury and improve their golf games. Kathy was the staff trainer at The International Golf Club in Bolton, Mass. from 2007-2011, and continues to offer golf fitness workshops to golfers of all abilities at golf clubs and gyms in Massachusetts. In addition to training athletes and fitness enthusiasts, Kathy coached high school lacrosse and field hockey for 13 years and currently officiates high school field hockey. She is also the co-author of a self help book for women entitled, *"Today's Superwoman- What to Do When Your Cape is at The Cleaner's"*. It is available on Amazon.

To contact Kathy for a free golf fitness consult, or to schedule an appointment, call 978-562-0377 or email her at kathy@personalbestpersonaltraining.com. Visit her website, www.personalbestpersonaltraining.com for free fitness tips and articles on nutrition, golf, yoga, strength training and more.

Pat Mullaly, is editor of GolfGurls.com, the Resource Site for Today's Woman Golfer and publisher of *Getting Golf Ready*. GolfGurls.com first appeared on the internet in 2009 and since has grown to include thousands of loyal followers. The blog offers golf tips especially for women golfers plus reviews on golf equipment, golf travel, golf fashions — everything related to the world of golf for women.

Pat has also authored several books on golf including "Putting Games,"
"Golf Journal" and "Golf Games, Golf Tournament Formats for Fun and Profit."